Pocket Manual of Community Health Nursing

Pocket Manual of Community Health Nursing

Maheswari Jaikumar
Principal
Miranda School and College of Nursing
Yelahanka, Bengaluru

JAYPEE BROTHERS MEDICAL PUBLISHERS
The Health Sciences Publisher
New Delhi | London

Jaypee Brothers Medical Publishers (P) Ltd

Headquarters
EMCA House
23/23-B, Ansari Road, Daryaganj
New Delhi 110 002, India
Landline: +91-11-23272143, +91-11-23272703
+91-11-23282021, +91-11-23245672
E-mail: jaypee@jaypeebrothers.com

Corporate Office
4838/24, Ansari Road, Daryaganj
New Delhi 110 002, India
Phone: +91-11-43574357
Fax: +91-11-43574314
E-mail: jaypee@jaypeebrothers.com

Overseas Office
J.P. Medical Ltd.
83, Victoria Street, London
SW1H 0HW (UK)
Phone: +44-20 3170 8910
E-mail: info@jpmedpub.com

EU GPSR Authorised Representative
Logos Europe, 9 rue Nicolas Poussin
17000, La Rochelle, France
Phone: +33 (0) 6 67 93 73 78
E-mail: contact@logoseurope.eu

Website: www.jaypeebrothers.com
Website: www.jaypeedigital.com

Inquiries for bulk sales may be solicited at: jaypee@jaypeebrothers.com

Pocket Manual of Community Health Nursing

First Edition: 2008

Reprint: **2026**

ISBN 978-81-8448-238-6

Printed in India

Preface to the Students

Dear learners,

This book is tailor made for you. To help get you involved in the study of this subject, a number of special features are incorporated throughout the book.

Topic boxes and tables are designed. These provide scientific information that would help you easily register and recollect the vital information as you render services.

Any exam causes anxiety; more so with a subject like community health. To help better prepare you for exam and comprehend the material, the information is provided in as capsules.

I hope that you enjoy the *Pocket Manual of Community Health Nursing* and that this book makes learning a rewarding process. Write to me and let me know how did you make out in your course.

Maheswari Jaikumar
(maheswari_jaikumar@yahoo.co.in)

Preface to the Instructors

A good book meets the needs of both instructors and students. Every teacher has a personal style and a philosophy of approach about teaching.

Considering this, I have chosen an eclectic approach to present the topics in a concrete information form. Pertinent information is present in clear definitions and tabular columns and boxes. Certain portions of the text accompany selected figures.

I wish that this book is of immense use to the instructors in the field of community health.

Maheswari Jaikumar

Acknowledgements

- At the outset, I wish to acknowledge and recognize the editorial team who have helped to make the textbook a reality.
- Heart felt gratitude to my parents Ganesan and Yamuna Ganesan for their love, support, compassion and commitment of life long learning.
- I wish to express my genuine gratitude to Mr. Jaikumar and my son Krethik Jaikumar for their sacrificial support.
- I am indebted to Ms. Manju in deciphering this manuscript into a reality.
- Last but not least, I bow down in reverence to the Lord Almighty, the source of all knowledge and wisdom for this unconditional blessings.

Contents

CHAPTER 1

Indicators of Health

THE FOLLOWING ARE THE INDICATORS OF HEALTH

1. Crude Birth Rate (CBR)
2. Crude Death Rate (CDR)
3. Specific Death Rate (SpDR)
4. Standardized Death Rate (SDR)
5. Proportional Mortality Rate
6. Age Proportional Mortality Rate
7. Maternal Mortality Rate (MMR)
8. Infant Mortality Rate (IMR)
9. Neonatal and Post Neonatal Mortality Rate
10. % of Low birth weight – babies (LBW)
11. Prenatal Mortality Rate
12. Pre-School Child Mortality Rate
13. Life Expectancy
14. Disability Days
15. Sullivan's Index
16. Physical Quality of Life Index
17. Disability Adjusted Life Years
18. Blindness Incidence Rate
19. Human Development Index

DEMOGRAPHIC PROFILE OF INDIA AS PER 2001 CENSUS

Sl No.	*Criteria*	*Rate/Picture*
1.	Population	1027,015,247
2.	Sex Ratio	933

Contd...

Contd...

Sl No.	*Criteria*		*Rate/Picture*
3.	Age Composition	0-4 yrs	12.6%
	5-14 yrs	27%	
	15-54 yrs	51.4%	
	55-64 yrs	5.2%	
	65 & above	3.8%	
4.	Density of Population		324 / Km^2
5.	Family Size		3.9
6.	Urban Population		25.7%
7.	Schedule Castes		16.5%
8.	Schedule Tribes		8.1%
9.	Literacy Rate	Female	54.2%
		Male	75.9%
		Total	65.4%
10.	Working Population		37.5%
11.	Crude Birth Rate (CBR)		26.6/1000 MYP – (1996)
12.	Crude Death Rate (CDR)		9/1000 MYP- (1996)
13.	Annual Growth Rate (AGR)		1.76%(94-96)
14.	Life Expectancy at Birth	Males	62.6 (94-96)
		Females	62.9(94-96)
15.	Probability of Dying Before 5th Birthday		0.095(1995)
16.	Infant Mortality Rate (IMR)		74/1000 LB (1996)
17.	Total Fertility Rate (TFR)		3.7('93-'95)
18.	Gross Reproduction Rate		2.14
19.	Population with Safe Drinking Water	Urban	85%

Contd...

Contd...

Sl No.	Criteria		Rate/Picture
		Rural	32%
		Combined	63%(1994)
20.	Excreta Disposal Facility		
		Urban	70% (1994)
		Rural	14% (1994)
		Combined	29% (1994)

MCH GOALS AND CURRENT LEVEL OF ACHIEVEMENT (INDIA)

No.	Indicator	Goals and target Current level	Ninth plan (2002)	National Population Policy 2000 (2010)
A	**Family Planning Indicators**			
	Crude Birth Rate	25.0 (2002)	23	21
	Total fertility rate	3.1 (2002)	2.6	2.1
	Couple protection rate	52 (2002)	60	Meet all Needs
B	**Mortality Indicators** per 1000			
	Infant Mortality	64 (2002)	50-56	<30
	Neonatal	45 (1999)	35	

Contd...

Contd...

No.	Indicator	Goals and target Current level	Ninth plan (2002)	National Population Policy 2000 (2010)
	Mortality			
	Under 5 Mortality	93 (2002)		
	MMR	4.07 (1998)	3	1
C	**Services (% coverage)**			
	Infants (Fully Immunized)	56 (2002)	65	100
	-Measles	67		
	-DPT	70		
	-Polio	70		
	-BCG	81		
	Pregnant women	82.9		
	TT			
	Antenatal Care	60 (1995-2002)	95	100
	Institutional Deliveries	34 (1998-99)	35	80
	Deliveries By Trained Personnel	42.3 (2000)	45	100
D	**Prevalence of Low Birth Weight Babies**	26 (1995-2000)	10	

Source: (7,77.78.79) and Annual Report (Govt. of India) 2003-2004

CHAPTER 2

Tools of Measurement in Community Health

2

I. Eyes and Ears of Public Health – or Tools of Measurement in Community are Rates, Ratios and Proportion.

A. **Rates :** Is obtained by the number of persons diagnosed as sick with the number of people examined, multiplied with a standard

E.g. Rate :

$$\frac{\text{Number Processing the...(Quantity)}}{\text{Total Individual Examined}} \times 1000$$

E.g. Death Rate :

$$\frac{\text{Number of Deaths in a Year}}{\text{Mid Year Population}} \times 1000$$

B. **Ratio:** Expresses a relation in size between two random quantities. The numerator is not a component of the demoninator

E.g. : X : Y (or) $\frac{X}{Y}$

$$\frac{\text{No. of individuals with Hypertension}}{\text{No. of individuals with Diabetes Mellitus}}$$

C. **Proportion :** is ratio that indicates the relation in magnitude of a part of the whole.

E.g. $$\frac{\text{No. of Children with diarrhoea in a village}}{\text{Total No. of Children of the same village}} \times 1000$$

D. Incidence Rate:

$$\frac{\text{No. of New Cases of X during the year}}{\text{Mid-Year population (MYP)}} \times 100$$

E. Prevalence

$$= \frac{\text{No. of New and Old cases of x}}{\text{Population Surveyed}} \times 100$$

MEASUREMENT IN COMMUNITY HEALTH

1. Measurement in Mortality- e.g. – IMR, MMR, NMR, U5MR, etc.
2. Measurement of Morbidity – e.g.: Incidence and prevalence of disease conditions in the society.
   E.g. : Incidence of TB
   Prevalence of Malaria
3. Measurements of Disability :
   E.g. : Disability Adjusted Life Years (DALY)
4. Measurement of Natality - E.g.: Birth Rate.
5. Measurement of Presence/Absence or distribution of the characteristics of the disease.
6. Measurement of Health Care Needs : E.g. :- Health Care Needs, utilization ratios, health–related events.
7. Measurement of the presence/absence of/ distributors of environmental or health related events.
8. Measurement of demographic variables.

Commonly Used Rates / Ratios

1. **Birth Rate (BR)**

$$\frac{\text{No. of live births during the year}}{\text{Estimated Mid Year Population}} \times 1000$$

2. **General Fertility Rate (GFR)**

$$\text{GFR} = \frac{\text{No. of live births in an area during the year}}{\text{Mid Year Female Population age 15-45 in the same area in the same year}} \times 1000$$

3. **General Marital Fertility Rate (GMFR)**

$$\text{GMFR} = \frac{\text{No. of live births}}{\text{Married Women in the reproductive age group in a given year}} \times 1000$$

4. **Age Specific Fertility Rate (ASFR)**

$$\text{ASFR} = \frac{\text{No. of live births in a year}}{\text{1000 married women in any specified age group}} \times 1000$$

5. **Total Fertility Rate (TFR)**

TFR = Is computed by adding ASFRs for all ages

6. **Gross Reproductive Rate (GRR)**

   GRR = Average No. of children that would beborn to married woman on experiencing the current fertility pattern throughout her reproductive span.

7. **Net Reproductive Rate (NRR)**

   NRR = Number of daughters a new born girl will bear during her life time assuming fixed age specific fertility and mortality rates

8. **Marriage Rate (MR)/Crude Marriage Rate (CMR)**

$$\text{CMR} = \frac{\text{No. of marriage in the year}}{\text{Mid. Year Population}} \times 1000$$

9. **Child Women Ratio**

$$\frac{\text{No. of children bearing age}}{\text{1000 women of child bearing age}}$$

(usually defined as 15-49 yrs of age)

10. **Abortion Rate (AR)**

    AR =

$$\frac{\text{No. of all types of abortion}}{\text{Total No. of Child bearing women}} \times 1000$$

11. **Abortion Ratio (AR)**

$$AR = \frac{\text{Abortions performed during a particular time period}}{\text{No. of live births over the same period}}$$

12. **Crude Death Rate (CDR)**

$$CDR = \frac{\text{Total no. of deaths in a given population in a specific period}}{\text{Total mid year population during the same period}} \times 1000$$

13. **Eligible Couples (EC)**
    EC = Refers to currently married couple, where in, the wife is in reproductive age of group (15-45 yrs of age) with one or two living children eligible for adoptions of fertility regulations methods (measure of contraception).
14. **Couple Protection Rate (CPR)**
    CPR = Percentage of eligible couples effectively protected against conception by one or the other approved methods of contraception (fertility regulation).
15. **Pre School Child Mortality Rate**

$$\frac{\text{Deaths in Children below 5 yrs}}{\text{Total Live Births}} \times 1000$$

16. **Life Expectancy:** Expected average life span of babies born, in a given year at a given place. It is calculated on the basis of age specific death rates existing at the time, on the assumption that the same rates will continue to prevail.
    - Average Life Expectancy – ALE (at birth) of X yrs
    - The higher the LE (at birth) the better the health status
17. **Disability Days:** The average number of days of disability per person.
18. **Sullivian's Index : L (SI)**

    SI = Life Expectancy at birth – disability days counted in years

    $$SI = LE\ (\text{at birth}) - \frac{\text{Disability days}}{365}$$
19. **Physical Quality of Life Index (PQLI)**
    - PQLI is a composite index.
    - It is based on weighted IMR, weighted Life Expectancy at age 1 and literacy.
    - The IMR weightage is on a scale 0 to 100. (0 for IMR of 229 / 1000 liver births, and 100 for 7 / 1000 live births)
    - Let the weighted IMR be X
    - The weightage of life expectancy at age 1 is on a scale 0 for 38 years to 100 for 77 years. Let it be 'Y'

- The Actual Literacy rate is considered. Let it be Z

$$\text{Then PQLI} = \frac{X + Y + Z}{3}$$

- PQLI varies from 0 (Worst) -50 (Avg.) -100 (Best)
- PQLI is used for ranking the countries according to human well being of their people.

20. **Quality Adjusted Life Years:** QALYs is used to assess the beneficial impact of two or more treatment modalities on and a specific disease.

    The following are the steps:

    1. Has the patient died following treatment
    2. Has he alternatively recovered?
    3. In the event of recovering, does he feel perfectly well.
    4. If so, a weight of 1 is given.
    5. Lesser weights are awarded, if he does not fully fit.
    6. The weights of each year of life gained from recovery following treatment are totalled to obtain QALY.

21. **Disability Adjusted Life Years:** The DALYs of a disease refers to measure of healthy years lost on account of one/or both of its unfavorable outcomes, namely death and dis-

ability. The impact of death depends on its timings.

The following contribute towards DALYs:

1. Severity of the disease
2. The time of the onset
3. The duration of the disease
4. Whether it ends in recovery or death

The following points, are useful in calculating DALY

1. Age specific morbidity and mortality rates
2. The proportion of its victims who develop isability
3. The mean age of onset of disability
4. The median duration of disability

   To assess the community burden of a disease, the DALYs of each one afflicted with are calculated and totalled.

HUMAN DEVELOPMENT INDEX

- The HDI (Human Development Index) is an indicator of human development of a country.
- It is an amalgamation of the following components:
  1. *A Long Life:* (measured by Life Expectation Index)
  2. *Knowledge:* (measured by enrolment ratio, in the school), and adult literacy rate

1. Combined Gross Enrolment Ratio : Ratio of children studying in schools : Total children of school going age.
2. Gross Enrolment : Is accorded 1/3rd weightage and adult literacy rate, 2/3rd weightage. The resulting value is called the "Education Index" (EI).

Decent Status of Living : Is measured by GDP per capita (i.e.).

$$\frac{\text{GDP}}{\text{Mid Year Population}}$$

GDP (Gross Domestic Product) : Refers to the value of all goods produced in a country, and all the services rendered in a given year.

- For international comparison, the GDP per capita is converted to American Dollars.
- The conversion is done taking into account the price level prevailing in the concerned country
- Following the conversion, GDP/capita is referred to as PPP. US$. (Purchasing Power Parity in American Dollars).
- GDP/capita is converted to GDP Index (GDPI).

CALCULATION OF INDICES

To calculate indices, the minimum (a) and maximum (b) goal post (values) are fixed as follows:

Goal Post for Calculating HDI

Goal post	*Life Expec-tancy At birth (yrs)*	*Combined Groups enrollment*	*Adult Literacy rate*	*GDP capita (US$)*
(a) Minimum	25	0	0	100
(b) Maximum	85	100	100	40,000

With respect to LEI and EI, use the following formula

Dimension Index =

$$\frac{\text{Actual Value} - \text{Minimum goal post}}{\text{Maximum goal post} - \text{Minimum goal post}}$$

GDP is calculated with log values

$$\text{GDPI} = \frac{\text{Log actual value} - \text{Log minimum goal post}}{\text{Log maximum goal post} - \text{Log minimum goal post}}$$

Calculation of HDI

HDI is calculated using the aforesaid three indices :

$$\text{HDI} = \frac{\text{LEI} + \text{EI} + \text{GDPI}}{3}$$

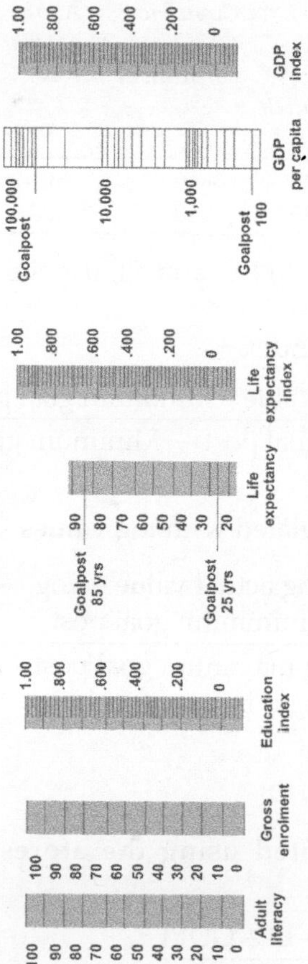

Calculation of Indices

- HDI varies from 0 to 1
- Developed countries have HDI >0.8
- Poorly developed countries have HDI < 0.5
- Moderately developed countries lies between these two cut-off points.

CHAPTER 3

Newborn Care

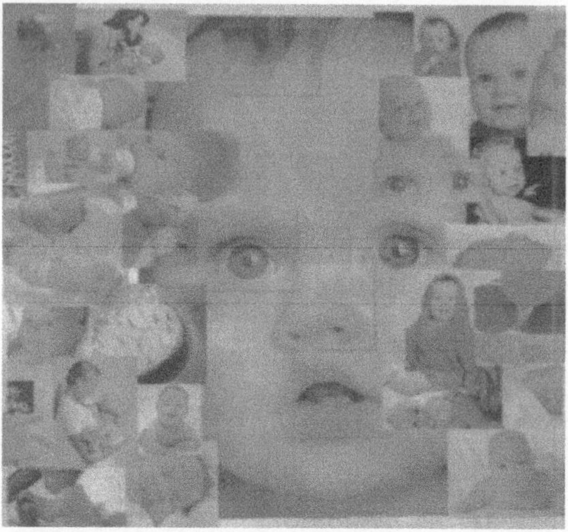

ESSENTIAL NEWBORN CARE (NB)

Refers to a set of care incorporating Newborn care at birth, provision of warmth, prevention of infection, care of Low Birth Weight Babies, sick newborns, and early identification of newborn requiring referral.

I. **Care at Birth :** Includes ensuring cleanliness of the following:
   1. Clean Hands
   2. Clean Surface
   3. Clean Scissors/Blade
   4. Clean Cord Tie
   5. Clean Cord Stumps

II. Provision of Warmth : Ensure the following:

1. Receive the NB at birth in a dry, prewarmed, clean cloth.
2. Place the baby under a warm source (200 Watt Bulb)
3. Dry the NB Immediately
4. Do not remove the vernix
5. Wrap and keep the baby warm
6. Place the baby close to the mother
7. Ensure a warm delivery room

III. Cord Care

1. Ensure that the umbilical cord is cut with a sterile scissors/blade
2. The cord is cut 2.5 cms from the abdomical skin surface.
3. Use sterile cord tie
4. Inspect the stump for bleeding.
5. If bleeding is present apply another cord tie
6. Leave the cord dry without antiseptics or dressing.

IV. Eye Care

1. Clean the eye with cotton swabs.
2. The eyes should be cleaned from medical to lateral
3. Do not use any prophylactic eye applications

V. Recording Birth Weight

1. Record the weight of the baby at birth using infant weighing scale.

VI. Initiation of Breastfeeding

1. Initiate breastfeeding within half-an hour following the delivery.
2. In case of caesarian section, the baby should be put to the breast, as soon as mother regains consciousness from anesthesia.

IMMEDIATE CARE OF THE NB

3

Aims at,

1. Establishment and maintenance of cardiopulmonary functions.
2. Resuscitation becomes necessary if natural breathing fails to establish within a minute.
3. Assess Apgar.

APGAR SCORING

Sign	*Score*		
	0	1	2
Heart Rate	Absent	Slow (<100 / min)	>100/min
Respiratory Effort	Absent	Slow irregular	Good/Crying

Contd...

Contd...

Sign	*Score*		
	0	1	2
Muscle Tone	Flaccid	Some flexion of the extremities	Active movements of the extremities
Reflex Response	No Response	Grimace	Cry
Color	Blue, Pale	Body pink Extremities – blue	Completely pink
Total Score 10	0-3	4-7	7-10

EXAMINATION OF NEWBORN AT BIRTH

Examine the NB as follows:

Sl No.	*Criteria*	*Intervention*
1	Malformations	• examine all the babies for malformations (Hydrocephalous, meningo-myeloclele, absence of annal opening)
2	Breathing Pattern	• assess the respiratory rate • normal RR – 30 – 40 breaths/ min • sometimes RR may go upto 60 • observe for the pattern of breathing

Contd...

Contd...

Sl No.	*Criteria*	*Intervention*
		• sometimes fast breathing is interspersed with slow breathing (Periodic Breathing). ABNORMAL BREATHING PATTERN includes the following • RR > 60/min • Presence of intercoastal/ subcoastal retractions • Associated apnoea, accompanied by cyanosis, • Heart rate - < 100 bpm
3	Heart Rate	• Normal HR – 100 – 160 bpm • Heart Rate <100, >160 are considered as abnormal
4	Perfusion gently apply pressure over the sole or sternum of the neonate using thumb and release to observe the time for refill of the capillaries	• Normal Capillary Refill Time < 3 Sec. • Capillary Refill is Prolonged in Shock/Hypotension and in Hypothermia
5	Colour	• The normal NB is pink • The baby appears pale in anemia • The baby appears yellow in Jaundice • The baby appears blue in cyanosis

PREVENTION OF HYPOTHERMIA

Hypothermia is a state in which the NB temperature is less than 36°C

Temperature recording	*Management*	*Prevention*
• Measure temperature using thermometer • Axillary/Rectal temp can be recorded • While recording rectal temperature, the thermometer should not be inserted more than 2 cm inside rectum • Temperature should be recorded for atleast 3 mins • Normal body temp = 36.5 to 37.5ºC.	• If the baby's temperature is less than 36°C, measure twice and confirm • Treat the hypothermic baby as follows • Warm the baby by placing under a heat source (i.e. 200 W bulb), placed 45 cm above the baby or use radiant warmer • Place the baby close to the mother • If the baby's condition do not improve, refer to FRU	• Keep the baby in close contact with the mother • Clothe the baby adequately, use woolen clothing if required • Maintain the room tem (where the baby is kept) • Keep the room free of draughts

PREVENTION OF INFECTION – NB

Prevent infection as/by following .....,

1. Administer TT immunization to the mother
2. Implement clean delivery practices
3. Ensure the cleanliness/and aseptic techniques of the personnel conducting the delivery
4. Use presterilized gloves for the conduct of delivery and while handling the baby
5. Cut the cord using sterile scissors/blade
6. Keep the cord dry
7. Do not use any antiseptics/dressing over the cord
8. Avoid pre lacteal feeds and water
9. Promote exclusive breastfeeding
10. Avoid bottle feeds
11. Prevent individuals with skin infections/ respiratory infections handling the baby
12. In case of institutional delivery administer zero dose OPV and BCG before the mother is discharged from the hospital.

CARE OF SICK NEWBORN

Illness and Severity	*Symptoms*	*Management*
I. MILD ILLNESS • Umbilical/ discharge • Conjunctivitis • Pyoderma II. SEVERE ILLNESS • Diarrhoea • Fast Breathing • Chest Indrawing • Decreased activity • Fever III. VERY SEVERE ILLNESS • Inability to feed • Persistent Hypothermia • Abdominal distension • Cyanosis • Apnoea • Convulsions • Bleeding • Severe • Jaundice • Grunting/ stridor	• Pus in the cord • Abnormal Secretions/ Crustations around the eye • Boils on skin surface • Respective symptoms	Mild illness can be treated at home • Apply gentian violet • Keep the area clean • Use clean clothes • Saline irrigation • Instillation of chloram-phenicol eye drops • Oral Antibiotics • Topical Applications of antiseptic creams • Antipyretics if presenting with fever • Ref Nsg care plan Diarrhoea • Ref to ARI care – Administer Oxygen

Contd...

Contd...

Illness and Severity	*Symptoms*	*Management*
		– Needs to be referred – Manage Appropriately 1. Ref to the health facilities 2. Before Ref/ transfer do the following – Administer 1st dose of antibiotic, IM (Inj Penicillin/ Ampicillin/ Gentamycin) – If convulsions are present Inj phenobarbitone IM–10 mg/kg – Send Ref slip – Arrange vehicle for transport – Mother should accompany the new born (if possible) Health educate to keep the baby warm during transport.

Contd...

NORMAL PHENOMENA AFTER BIRTH

Certain adaptive changes take place in an NB after birth during the 1st week. These changes are termed as NORMAL PHENOMENA. These are not pathological. They are as follows:

Sl. No.	*Phenomena*	*Description*
1.	Meconium passage	• Meconium is the first stool of newborn. • It is dark, greenish black and sticky in nature • Meconium is made up of intrauterine swallowed amniotic fluid, intestinal secretions and shed epithelial cells. • Meconium is first passed within 24 hrs of birth • Some fetus pass *in utero* • Non passage of meconium is a cause for concern (may suggest imperforation, intestinal obstruction. Such case should be referred.
2.	Passage of urine	• Newborns usually pass urine in the delivery room soon after the birth • (or) with 24-48 hrs • non-passage of urine within 48 hrs is abnormal and requires referral.

Contd...

Contd...

Sl. No.	*Phenomena*	*Description*
		• A normal NB would pass urine 6-7 times/day (after 2nd day) • Some NB may cry just before passage of urine (this is normal)
3.	Transitional stools	• Following the passage of meconium, the NB continues, to pass dark, greenish, sticky stools, 3-4 times/day for the next 2-3 days • This is followed by change in the characteristic of the stool. • This is termed as transitional stool The features of the transitional stool are as : – The stool is greenish yellow – Increased frequency of stools (upto 15 times/day) – Loose watery consistency – This may last from 6 to 20 days – Re-assure the mother – After 2 weeks, the neonate may pass upto 15-20 stools/ day (this may follow every feeding session) or

Contd...

Contd...

Sl. No.	*Phenomena*	*Description*
		– The child may pass once in 5-6 days (In case of diarrhea, stool may have associated blood/mucus, is and associated with dehydration) – When NB passes stools once in 5-6 days it may be normal, (when the stool is yellow, soft, there is no abdominal destention (or) yellow coloured vomitus)
4.	Vomiting	• Some NB frequently vomit mucoid secretions during the first day • This is due to swallowed amniotic fluid • If the baby is not properly burped, after a feed the baby may re-gurgiate/vomit the feed. • Abnormal vomiting is present in case of intestinal obstruction (in such cases, vomiting in persistent bile or blood stained and projectile in nature.
5.	Mongolian spot	• Are bluish-black patches of pigmentation especially over the sacral and buttock areas. • Mongollian spots may also be seen in trunk and extremities.

Contd...

Contd...

Sl. No.	*Phenomena*	*Description*
		• The pigmentation will disappear by 6 months of age
6.	Erythema toxicum	• Erythematous rash may appear on the 2nd or 3rd day • It begins from the face and spreads to the trunk, extremities, over next 24 hrs. It disappears spontaneously within 2-3 days
7.	Vaginal discharge and bleeding	• Female babies have thin white mucoid secretions from vagina. • Clean the secretion with water and keep the place dry. • Pseudo menstruation (withdrawal bleeding) occurs in few babies after 3-5 days. • Keep the genitalia clean and dry
8.	Mastitis	• Breast engorgement may occur on the third or the fourth day. • This phenomenon is due to transplacental transfer of the maternal hormones • Local massage, formentation or manual expression of discharge must be avoided • Re-assure the mother

Contd...

3

Contd...

Sl. No.	*Phenomena*	*Description*
9.	Physiological jaundice	• Refers to jaundice appearing after 24 hrs of birth • Peak level of bilirubin exceeds upto 15 mg/dl. • Jaundice decreases by 7-10 days of life. • High levels of bilirubin >20 mg/dl are associated with risk of brain damage
10.	Catput/Cephalo-hematoma	• Some babies have biggy swelling over the scalp (CATPUT SUCCEDANEUM) • This is due to pressure over the presenting part. • Cephalohematoma (Sub peri-osteal haemorrhage) appears after 2-3 days • Cephalohematoma is usually associated with anemia or jaundice.
11.	Hydrocephalus	• Requires Medical Intervention

CARE OF LOW BIRTH WEIGHT BABIES

Definition : LBW babies refers to babies whose birth weight is < 2500 gm (2.5 kg) at birth

LBW Babies :
- Pre-Term Babies (Born before 37 wks of gestation)
- IUGR (Full term Intra-uterine growth retardation or SFD = Small for Date Babies)

Physical Examination of LBW Babies Reveals

1. Absence of sole creases.
2. Or present only in the anterior 1/3 of the sole
3. The breast nodule is less the <5 mm in diameter.
4. The ear does not re-coil immediately on folding.
5. The hair are fine and wooly.
6. In male infants the testis is not fully descended into the scrotum, and in female babies the vaginal opening is exposed and clitoris is prominent.

Management of LBW Babies : Focus on the following:

1. Prevention of Hypothermia
2. Promotion of exclusive breastfeeding
3. Prevention of infection

Resuscitation of Newborn

(Not Breathing soon after birth)

- Take steps to resuscitate the baby

Equipment Needed for Neonatal Resuscitation

- Self–Inflating Bag and Mask
- Oxygen
- Mucus sucker
- Syringe/needle (no. 24)
- Adrenaline (1:1000 dil)

MANAGEMENT OF LBW BABIES

Sl. No.	*Problem*	*Management*
1.	Hypothermia	• Room in the baby with the mother • Advocate skin to skin contact • Cloth the baby adequately use woolen clothes if required • Keep the baby warm and dry • The room where the baby is kept should be kept warm free from cold draughts • Provide additional heat to the baby by using heat source (100-200 W bulb placed 18″ from the baby • Record the temperature of the baby every 3-4 hrs to ensure optimal temp maintenance
2.	Feeding	• Promote and insist only on breastfeeding

Contd...

Contd...

Sl. No.	*Problem*	*Management*
		• Avoid/Discourage pre lacteal feeds • Initiate breastfeeding as early as possible • In instances where the baby is not able to suck at the breast, breast milk can be expressed into a clean vessel and feed using cup and spoon • Discourage the use of bottles for feeding • Adequacy of feeding can be ascertained by baby's weight gain (after a week the baby is expected to gain about 15-20 gm/day or 100-140 gm (wk)
3.	Prevention of Infection	• Discourage and prevent individuals with diarrhea/respiratory conditions handling the baby • The mother and care takers should wash their hands using soap before handling the baby • Advice the mother/care taker to use mask to avoid droplet infection • Avoid pre-lacteal feeds and water

Contd...

Contd...

Sl. No.	*Problem*	*Management*
		• The surrounding environment where the baby is kept should be dry and clean • Follow and adhere to the recommended immunization schedule • The dose of vaccine is same as for normal babies
4.	Any Other Problems (or) Complications	• Ref to FRU

CHAPTER 4

Breast Feeding

Breast Milk is the nature's gift to the baby. Breast Feeding is the fundamental right of the baby. An average Indian mother secretes 450-600 ml of milk daily with 12.9% protein.

Exclusive Breast Feeding refers to feeding the child with only breast milk, no other food/fluid.

Colostrum refers to the first secretion from the breast usually serous, light yellowish in colour, colotrum is rich in immunoglobulin, and therefore, potently provides protection against disease.

Pre-Lacteal Feeds refers to any feed introduced (e.g. Water, Honey, Donkey's Milk, Cow's Milk, etc.) before the introduction of colostrum or breast milk to the baby.

Advantages of Breast Feeding

1. Natural and convenient
2. It contains the requisite nutrition for the baby
3. It easily digestible and assimilable
4. Breast feeding is economical, readily available
5. It prevents infections
6. Promotes mother baby bonding
7. Promotes optimal growth and development (Physical, Intellectual)

8. Prevents malnutrition
9. Helps in early involution of the uterus
10. Breast feeding helps to delay the birth of subsequent child.

Initiation of Breast Feeding

1. *In case of normal delivery:* as early as possible
2. *In case of cesarean section:* as early as possible; as soon as the mother recovers from anesthesia.

Frequency and Duration of Breast Feeding

1. Advice breast feeding on demand
2. The baby should be put to breast as long as it wants
3. Feed the baby on both breast (if the baby refuses) as it would feel full with milk from the breast, then for the next feed, feed the baby on the other breast.
4. Encourage a complete feed on one breast, so that the child gets (fore and Hind Milk)
5. Discourage Bottle feeding.

Common Problems – During Breast Feeding

1. Flat – or retracted nipple
2. Sore nipple
3. Engorged breast, mastitis, breast abscess.

Duration Breast Feeding

1. Exclusive breast feeding should be advocated for 6 months
2. There after the child should be weaned gradually and complementary feeds should be introduced
3. Breast feeding can be continued as long as desired along with complementary foods
4. When the mother decides to stop breast feeding care should be taken to stop gradually.

CONTENTS OF BREAST MILK

Sl. No.	*Constituents*	*Qty. gms / Lt*
1.	**Proteins**	11
	• Casein	4
	• Soluble Proteins	7
	• Lactalbumin	3.5
	• B. Lactoglobulin	0
	• Lactotrasferrin	1-2
	• Immunoglobulin	1-2
	• Lysosome	0.5
2.	**Non-Protein Lipids**	
	• Linolenic acid	3.5
3.	**Carbohydrates :**	
	• Lactose	70
	• Nitrogenous	62
	• Oligosaccharides	8

Contd...

Contd...

Sl. No.		*Constituents*	*Qty. gms / Lt*
4.		**Minerals**	
	–	Ca	0.33
	–	P	0.15
	–	Fe	0.4-1.5 mg
5.		**Vitamins**	
	–	C	60 mg
	–	D	50 1U
6		**Energy**	640-720 Kcal/2670-3000 KJ (i.e.) the energy value/per 100 ml = 70 kcal

NUTRITIONAL REQUIREMENT – INFANT

Sl. No.	*Item*	*First 6 Mo*	*Second 6 Mo*
1.	Energy	120 kcal/ kg wt	100 kcal /kg
2.	Proteins	2.4 gm milk protein/kg wt	1.8 – 1.2 G/kg
3.	Carbohydrates	10 G / kg	10 G/kg
4.	Fats	5 G/kg	5 G/kg
5.	Calcium	500 – 600 mg	500 – 600 mg
6.	Iron	1 mg/kg	1 mg/kg
7.	Vit 'A'	400 µ of retinol	300 microgram of retinol
8.	Vit ' C '	30 mg	30 mg

Contd...

Contd...

Sl. No.	Item	First 6 Mo	Second 6 Mo
9.	Vit 'D'	200 IU	200 IU
10.	Folates	25 Microgram	25 Microgram
11.	Cyanoco-balamine	0.2 Microgram	0.2 Microgram

CHAPTER 5

Complementary Feeding and Growth Monitoring

Complementary Feeding refers to introduction of semisolid feeding for infants at 6 months age in addition to breast feeding.

RATIONALE

Six months is considered to be ideal to start complementary feeding due to the following:

1. The baby's growth and development is rapid and the baby needs additional food and water to meet the growing need if not the baby will develop malnutrition.
2. By six months, the baby's activity increases and hence, BMR is high
3. Baby's GI system is ready to digest semisolid foods
4. Baby has good appetite and accepts food readily
5. The breast milk secretion starts declining slowly.

Principles of Complementary Feeding

1. Introduce one food/Item at a time
2. Start with clear fluids, and then semisolids
3. Start with small Quantity (1 tsp) and increase gradually
4. Initially introduce complementary foods between feeds

5. Use spoon, cup, etc. for feeding (avoid bottle feeding).

Advocated Frequency

Sl. No.	*Age*	*Frequency of Feeds*
1	5-6 Mo.	2-3 times/day
2	7-9 Mo.	3-4 times/day
3	10-11 Mo.	4-5 times/day
4	1 Yr.	5-6 times/day

Applied Aspects of Complementary Feeding

1. Start Complementary feeding between 4 and 6 Month,
2. Continue Breast Feeding as long as possible
3. Give as much as the baby wants at a time
4. Give easily available home cooked foods
5. Feeding can be continued during illness
6. Use minimum water for cooking and mash the food
7. Wash hands before cooking and feeding
8. Keep foods covered
9. Advocate a mixed balanced diet suiting to the socioeconomic status
10. The semisolid foods should have high caloric value, easily digestible, palatable, inexpensive and with low viscosity.

GUIDELINES FOR COMPLEMENTARY FEEDING

Sl No.	*Age*	*Guidelines for feeding*
1.	6-12 Months	1. Mash all the foods 2. Give semisolid foods 3. Start with 1 or 2 tsp 4. Increase the amount gradually 5. Increase the variety of food gradually 6. Advocate foods routinely cooked at home 7. Avoid the usage of feeding bottles
2.	12 – 24 Months	1. The infant – needs 1000 kcal – 1500 kcals 2. The Mother may continue breast feeding 3. Avoid spicy foods 4. Offer food at least five times a day
3.	> 24 Months and older	1. Advice family food for three times a day 2. Give extra food if the child prefers

5

SUGGESTED COMPLIMENTARY FEEDS

Sl No.	*Age*	*Type of feed*	*Suggested feed*
1.	0-4 Mo.	Fluids	• Breast milk
2.	5 Mo.	Fluids 150-200 ml/ feeds	• Nestum rice • Farex • Lactogen I • Tender coconut water • Mashed dhal water • Rice water • Fruit juices – very cleanly prepared • Vegetable soups
3.	6 Mo.	Soft semi-solids 200-225 ml/ feed	• Idli paste (water consistency) • Idiappam (paste) • Manna (Ragi Malt) • Beaten rice • Mashed vegetables and fruits • Lactogen II
4.	7 Mo.	Semisolids 225-250 ml/ feed	• As stated above • Increase the quantity and consistency
5.	8 Mo.	Solids 250-275 ml/ feed	• Beaten and mashed preparations • Increase the quantity and consistency

Contd...

Contd...

Sl No.	Age	Type of feed	Suggested feed
6.	9 Mo.	Solids	• Ingredients as stated above
		300 ml/feed	• Increase the quantity • Feed every 3-4 hrs
7.	10 Mo.	Solids	• Feed depending the likes of the child
8.	10-12 Mo.	Solids	• Adult's diet with little alteration according to intake

NOTE : Milk to be continued at all stages.

5

POINTS TO REMEMBER – WEANING PROCESS

1. Do not force feeds
2. Do not over feed
3. Try new preparations- introduce very small quantities initially
4. Introduce only one new item in a week
5. Always observe the child's reaction to new feed, his likeliness and motion, signs of allergy
6. Never give any thing raw except for plantain
7. Prepare infant food with utmost cleanliness
8. Dry all feeding items in broad sunlight after a thorough wash (for a minimum of 2 hours)
9. Try to avoid bottle feeds

10. Do not give any tinned food or foods with preservations
11. Add iodized salt to infant foods while preparing
12. Immunize duely
13. Weigh the child every month on specified day, e.g. 24th of every month
14. Always consult a doctor. If you suspect any thing wrong or suspicion arises
15. Always have paracetamol drops at home
16. Never put the child on medication without doctors prescription.

GROWTH MONITORING

Def: Refers to the assessment of the nutritional status of the child, by using road to health chart

- Growth Monitoring is an operational strategy to promote health and
- Serves as practical of guidance to ensure regular growth

Objective of Growth Monitoring

1. Detect growth faltering at the earliest.
2. Promote satisfactory growth by appropriate intervention.
3. Create awareness on growth and the importance of monitoring among mothers.
4. Identify 'at risk' for malnutrition children and implement relevant intervention.

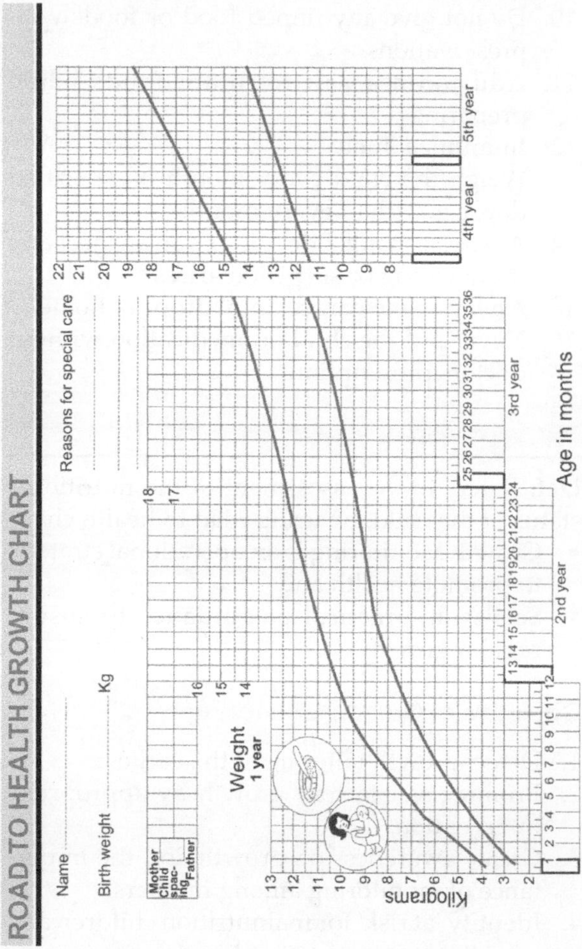
ROAD TO HEALTH GROWTH CHART
Name
Birth weight Kg
Reasons for special care
Mother Child spacing Father
Weight
1 year
Kilograms
2nd year
3rd year
4th year
5th year
Age in months

GROWTH MONITORING ON A GROWTH CHART

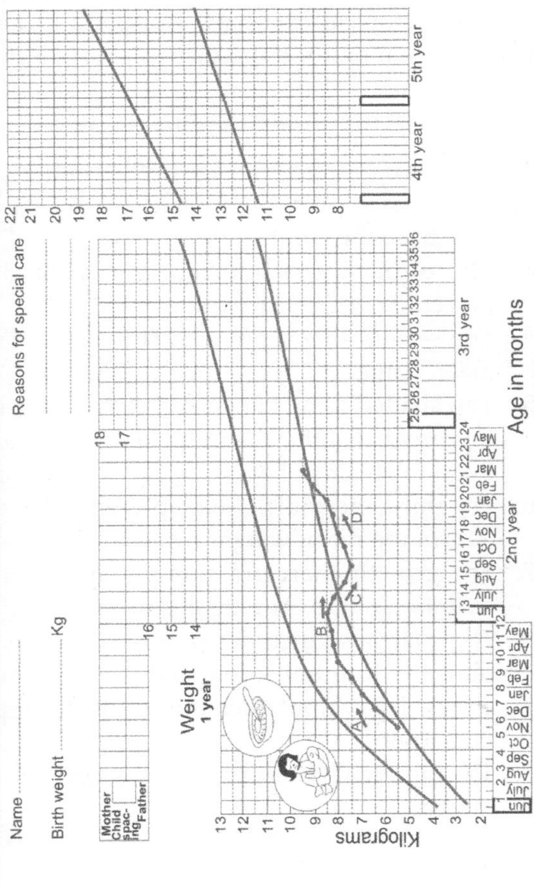

Tool to Monitor the Growth

"The Road the Health Chart" is a specially designed card to monitor the growth status of a child.

Contents of the Growth Chart

1. The X axis records the age of the child.
2. The Y axis provides means to record the weight of the child.
3. The upper most line represents the 50th percentile of the Harvard standard.
4. The second line represents 80% of the same mean value.
5. The shaded zone between the aforesaid line represent Healthy Zone and hence, termed as Road to Health Chart.
6. The third and fourth line represents 70% and 60% of the mean weight respectively.
7. The growth chart presents a graphic representation of the growth of the child.
8. The chart also includes provisions for recording the immunization, status, deworming status, Iron supplementation, Vit A supplementation.
9. The growth chart serves as a complete health record.

Uses of Growth Chart

1. Helps in growth monitoring.
2. Serves as diagnostic tool for identifying growth faltering and high risk children.
3. Helps in planning and policy making.
4. Serves as an educational tool.
5. Serves as tool for action.
6. Helps in evaluating the corrective measures taken in case of nutritional rehabilitation as required.
7. Serves as a tool for teaching.

MILESTONES OF DEVELOPMENT

Age	*Motor Development*	*Language Development*	*Adaptive Development*	*Socio-personal Development*
6-8 Wks	—	—	—	Looks at the mother and smiles
3 Mo.	Holds Head erect	—	—	—
4-5 Mo.	—	Listening	Begins to reach out for objects	Recognizes mother
6-8 Mo.	Sits without support	Experimentation of with noises	Transfers objects hand to hand	Enjoys hide and seek

Contd...

Contd...

Age	*Motor Development*	*Language Development*	*Adaptive Development*	*Socio-personal Development*
9-10 Mo.	Crawling	Increasing range of sounds	Releases objects	Suspicious of strangers
10-11 Mo.	Stands with support	First words	—	—
12-14 Mo.	Walks wide base	—	Builds	—
18-21 Mo.	Walks narrow base beginning to run	Joining words together	Beginning to explore	—
24 Mo.	Runs	Short sentences	—	Day by Day

THE ROLE OF A COMMUNITY HEALTH WORKER IN THE CARE OF CHILDREN

The community health worker will ensure and promote the following:

- Ensure the marriageable age of female to be 21 years and for boys to be 24 years

- Register all confirmed cases of pregnancy within 3 months (Ideally 10 wks)
- Ensure a minimum of five antenatal visits, subjecting them to antenatal examinations
- Education to antenatal mothers on the importance of diet, sleep and exercise (allied household works)
- Refer cases requiring specialist services
- Promoting institutional deliveries
- Promoting breast feeding within half an hour of birth in case of natural delivery and as early as possible in case of delivery by caesarian section
- Discourage pre-lacteal feeds (such as donkey's milk, honey, sugar water, etc.)
- Promoting exclusive breast feeding (EBF for a minimum of 4 months and gradual wearing following four months
- Weigh the baby as soon as it is born and to weigh the baby periodically every month
- Promote nutritional supplementation if the child is found underweight
- Ensure a complete immunization status for all under fives (ref National Immunization Schedule)
- Training mothers on the home management of diarrhoea and ARI
- Promote general hygiene and food hygiene to mothers and to all the family members.

CHAPTER 6

Anthropometry: U5 Children

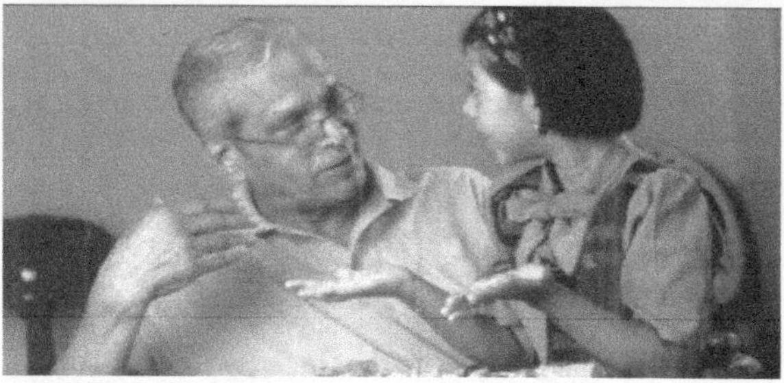

6

Anthropometry is the process of recording/ monitoring Ht, Wt, Skin fold thickness, head circumference, chest circumference, etc. It indicates valuable information on the nutritional status of the child.

Anthropometrics recorded and monitored over a period will serve as powerful tool, to reflect the growth and development pattern of the children.

ANTHROPOMETRY U5 CHILDREN AVERAGE WEIGHT / HEIGHT INCREASE (0-5 YRS)

Age	*Increments*
	Weight Increments/wk
0-3 months	200 gms
4-6 months	150 gms
7-9 months	100 gms
10-12 months	50-75 gms

Contd...

Contd...

Age	*Increments*
	Weight Increments/yr
1-2 yrs	2.5 kgs
3-5 yrs	2 kgs
	Length increments/yr
1st Year	25 cms
2nd Year	12 cms
3rd Year	9 cms
4th Year	7 cms
5th Year	6 cms

FORMULA TO CALCULATE WT/HT

1. The average birth weight of the child in Indian context – 2.7 kg – 2.9 kg
2. 3 Mo – 1 Yr = $\frac{\text{Age in Months} + 9}{2}$ (Wt in kgs)

   (OR)

   Age in months + 11 (Wt in lbs)
3. 1-6 Yrs = Age in yrs × 2 + 8 = Wt in kgs

   (OR)

   Age in yrs × 5 + 17 = Wt in lbs
4. 7–12 Yrs = $\frac{\text{Age in yrs} \times 7 - 5}{2}$ Wt in kgs

   (OR)

   Age in yrs × 7 + 5 = Wt in lbs
5. Formula to Calculate Ht

   2-12 yrs = Age in yrs × 6 +77

(OR)

Age in yrs × 2.5 + 30 length in inches

Adults

1. Expected Weight = Ht in cm – 100 × 0.9

INTERPRETATION OF INDICATORS

$$\text{Weight/Height \%} = \frac{\text{Weight of the child}}{\text{Weight of a normal child at same height}} \times 100$$

6

$$\text{Height/age \%} = \frac{\text{Height of the child}}{\text{Height of a normal child at same age}} \times 100$$

Nutritional Status	*Stunting (% of height/ age)*	*Wasting (% of weight/ height)*
Normal	> 95	> 90
Mildly impaired	87.5 -95	80-90
Moderately impaired	80-87.5	70-80
Severely impaired	< 80	< 70

Chest Circumference (CC): Is measured by placing

1. The tape at the level of the nipple in a plane at right angle to the spine.
2. Record the measurement in mid respiration.

Measurements

Sl. No.	*Age*	*Measurement (cm)*
1	At Birth	30-32
2	1 Yr	The CC is almost equal to HC
3	1 year and thereafter	CC exceeds HC gradually
4	By 5 yrs	CC is 5 cm more than HC

Applied Aspects

1. Head Circumference (HC) at birth : 34 cms
2. Chest Circumference (CC) at birth : 32 cms
3. At End of 1 yr : HC and CC equals
4. After 1 yr : CC over takes HC
5. In severely malnourished children overtaking may be delayed by 3-4 yrs

In vitamin D Deficiency (Pigeon Chest) CC is abnormal

HEAD CIRCUMFERENCE (HC) NORMAL FINDINGS

Sl. No.	*Age*	*HC in CMS*
1.	At birth	33-35
2.	3 months	40
3.	6 months	43
4.	1 Yr	45
5.	2 Yrs	48
6.	7 Yrs	50
7.	12 Yrs	52
8.	18 Yrs	55

Procedure for measuring Head Circumference

Measure the head at its greatest circumference usually above the eyes, brows and pinna of he ears and around the occipital prominence.

Articles Required

1. Inch Tape
2. Paper/Pencil/Pen for recording

There will be alteration in certain conditions like hydrocephalous, Microcephalus, Anencephaly, Cephalhematoma, etc.

SKIN FOLD THICKNESS AND MID ARM CIRCUMFERENCE

Skin Fold Thickness

1. Is the measurement of body fat
2. Is measured using special device – calipers
3. The most common sites are triceps, subscapular, supra iliac, abdomen and upper thigh.

Mid Arm Circumference (MAC) for U5 Children

1. MAC is an indirect measure of muscle mass.
2. MAC is measured at mid point from the acromion process and the olecranon process
3. MAC helps in identifying under nutrition among children
4. Values less than 12.5 indicate significant wasting and under nutrition.
5. MAC is indicated for children more than 1 yr
6. MAC is usually measured in the non-dominant hand (well developed muscle of dominant hand will interfere with accurate reading).

CHAPTER 7

Immunization

7

Immunization or Vaccination in given to prevent Vaccine Preventable Diseases (VPD) and is the most important step in implementing primordial/ Primary Prevention strategies among under fives.

THE NATIONAL IMMUNIZATION SCHEDULE

Sl. No.	*Vaccine*	*Age*	*Dose*	*Route*	*Site*
1.	TT	Pregnant Women Children	0.5 ml	I M	Deltoid
2.	BCG (Bacille Calmette-Guérin)	At Birth 6 Wks	0.05 ml 0.1 ml	ID ID	Upper arm Deltoid
3.	OPV (Oral Polio Vaccine)	At Birth (Zero Polio) 6 Wks 10 Wks 14 Wks	2 Drops	Oral	Oral
4.	DPT (Diphtheria) Pertussis Tetanus	6 Wks 10 Wks 14 Wks	0.5 ml 0.5 ml	IM	Antero-lateral aspect of thigh
5.	Measles	On Completing 9 Months	0.5 ml	IM/SC	Deltoid, Antero-lateral aspect of thigh

Contd...

Contd...

Sl. No.	*Vaccine*	*Age*	*Dose*	*Route*	*Site*
6.	DPTI Booster	16-24 Months or 12 Months after the III dose	0.5 ml	IM	Antero-lateral aspect of thigh
7.	OPVI Booster	16-24 Months	2 Drops	Oral	Oral
8.	DT (Diphtheria, Tetanus)	5 yrs	0.5 ml	IM	Deltoid
9.	TT (Tetanus Toxoid)	10 Yrs	0.5 ml	IM	Deltoid
		16 Yrs	0.5 ml	IM	Deltoid

IM–Intramuscular; ID–Intradermal; SC–Subcutaneous

- TT (2) doses are given to pregnant women
  - I Dose TT – on First contact
  - II Dose TT – 1 Month following I dose
  - One dose of TT is enough if the woman conceives within 3 yrs following the previous pregnancy.
- Once vial is opened it should be promptly used/discarded (Especially BCG Vaccine).
- Malnutrition, low of grade fever, mild respiratory infections, diarrhoea, minor illness are not contraindications to immunization
- BCG vaccine must be used as early as possible after dissolving.

SUGGESTED IMMUNIZATION SCHEDULE FROM BIRTH TO 16 YRS (INCL OPTIONAL VACCINES)

Sl. No.	Recommended Age	Vaccine	Dose	Disease Preventable	Type of Vaccine	Dosage	Route
1.	Birth to 2 wks	BCG	1	Tuberculosis	Live attenuated vaccine	0.1 ml	ID
2.	Birth to 2 wks	OPV	0 (1)	Poliomyelitis	Live attenuated vaccine	2 drops	Oral
3.	Birth to 2 wks	HBV	1	Hepatitis	Recombinant surface Antigen Protein	0.5 ml 1 ml	IM
4.	6 Weeks	DPT	1	Diphtheria Pertussis Tetanus	Inactivated or Killed Vaccine	0.5 ml	IM
5.	6 Weeks	OPV	2	Polio	Live attenuated	2 drops	Oral
6.	6 Weeks	HBV	2	As aforesaid	As aforesaid	1 ml	IM.
7.	6 Weeks	HIB	1	H. influenza B. meningitis	Inactivated or Killed Vaccine	0.5 ml	IM
8.	10 Weeks	DPT	2	As aforesaid	As aforesaid	0.5 ml	IM

Contd...

Contd...

Sl. No.	*Recommended Age*	*Vaccine*	*Dose*	*Disease Preventable*	*Type of Vaccine*	*Dosage*	*Route*
9.	10 Weeks	OPV	3	As aforesaid	As aforesaid	0.5 ml	IM
10.	10 Weeks	HIB	2	As aforesaid	As aforesaid	0.5 ml	IM
HBV–Hepatitis B Vaccine							
11.	14 Weeks	DPT	3	As aforesaid	As aforesaid	0.5 ml	IM
12.		OPV	4	As aforesaid	As aforesaid	0.5 ml	IM
13.		HIB	3	As aforesaid	As aforesaid	0.5 ml	IM
14.		HBV	3	As aforesaid	As aforesaid	0.5 ml	IM
15.	6 Months	Oral Vit 'A'	–	Vit 'A' Deficiency	–	1 lack IU	Oral
16.	10 Months	Measles	1	Measles	Live attenuated vaccine	0.5 ml	SC
17.	15 Months	MMR	1	Mumps, Measles, Rubella	Live attenuated vaccine	0.5 ml	SC
18.	> 1 yr	Varicella vaccine	-	Chicken pox	Live attenuated vaccine	0.5 ml	SC
19.	18 Months	HIB	Booster	As aforestated	As aforestated	0.5 ml	IM

Contd...

Contd...

Sl. No.	Recommended Age	Vaccine	Dose	Disease Preventable	Type of Vaccine	Dosage	Route
20.		DPT	B1	As aforestated	As aforestated		IM
21.		OPV	B1	As aforestated	As aforestated		Oral
22.	2 yrs	Typhoid Vaccine	Repeat in 3 yrs	Typhoid	Live attenuated vaccine	0.5 ml	IM
23.	>2 yrs	HAV	1	Hepatitis A	Live attenuated vaccine	0.5 ml	IM
24.	5 yrs	HAV	2	As stated above	As aforestated	0.5 ml	IM
25.	5 yrs	DT	B2	Diphtheria Tetanus	Toxoid	0.5 ml	IM
26.	5 yrs	OPV	B2	As stated above	As aforestated	–	Oral
27.	10 yrs	TT	B3	Tetanus	Toxoid	0.5 ml	IM
28.	16 yrs	TT	B3	As stated above	Toxoid		IM
29.	Under 5 pulse polio prog.	OPV	–	Polio	Live attenuated vaccine	2 drops	Oral

B1–Booster-1 B2–Booster-2
B3–Booster 3 HAV–Hepatitis A Vaccine

POTENTIAL ADVERSE REACTIONS FOLLOWING IMMUNIZATION

Sl. No.	*Vaccine*	*Adverse Reactions*	*Symptoms*	*Management*
1.	Any vaccine	Anaphylaxis (extremely rare)	Within few minutes • Acute decompensation of circulatory system • Hypovolumic shock • Altered sensorium • Laryngospasm/oedema • Acute respiratory distress	• Adrenaline (1:10,000) • Dose – 0.01ml /kg body wt SC/IM immediately • CPR • IV volume expanders • O_2 inhalation • Hypovolumic Inj IV
2.	DTP	Hypotensive, Hyporesponsive episode (rare)	Within 12 hrs • Acute paleness • Transient loss of consciousness	• IV fluids • Dexamethasone • O_2
3.	DPT	Incessant cry	Within 48-72 hrs	• Sedation • Analgesic • Feeding advice

Contd...

Contd...

Sl. No.	*Vaccine*	*Adverse Reactions*	*Symptoms*	*Management*
				• Avoid DPT subsequent dose • Administer DT
4.	BCG	Lymphadenitis local ulcer	Within 2-6 Mo • Firm to soft axillary lymphadenitis • Ulcer at the site of injection	• If soft fluid aspiration give INH 5 mgm/kg once daily for 5 months
5.	Any Vaccine	• Bacterial abscess • Sciatic nerve injury	Within 72 hrs, fluctuant or firm abscess with or without fever	• Antibiotic • Antipyretics • Drainage if needed
6.	DPT, DT, TT Typhoid and HB	Sterile abscess	By 72 hrs • Minimum inflammation • No fever	Drainage if needed
7.	DPT, Measles	Hyper – pyrexia	By 12-24 hrs	• Antipyretics • Tepid water sponging
8.	Any vaccine	Hyper – pyrexia	By 12-24 hrs	• Antipyretics

EPIDEMIOLOGICAL FEATURES OF VACCINE PREVENTABLE DISEASES

Disease	*Causative agent*	*Mode of transmission*	*Reservoir*	*Incubation period*	*Communicability*	*Major complications*	*Specific treatment*	*Immunity*
Poliomyelitis	Polio viruses types I,II and III	Faecally-contaminated material pharyngeal secretions	Man	7-14 days (range 3-25 days)	First week before & after onset of symptoms (range 3-6 weeks)	Residual paralysis of limbs, paralysis of respiratory muscles can lead to death	None	Type specific lifelong

Contd...

Contd...

Disease	*Causative agent*	*Mode of transmission*	*Reservoir*	*Incubation period*	*Communicability*	*Major complications*	*Specific treatment*	*Immunity*
Measles	Mealses virus	Air-borne direct contact with nasal or throat secretions	Man	8-13 days	Slightly before prodromal period to 4 days after rash	Diarrhea Pneumonia Otitis media Conjunctivitis Encephalitis, Malnutrition	None	Life-long
Diphtheria	*Corynebacterium diphtheriae*	Air-borne Direct contact	Man	2-5 days	2 weeks or less	Respiratory obstruction myocarditis nerve palsy	20,000-100,000 units of antitoxin and antibiotics	Clinical disease may not provide life-long immunity

Contd...

Contd...

Disease	*Causative agent*	*Mode of transmission*	*Reservoir*	*Incubation period*	*Communicability*	*Major complications*	*Specific treatment*	*Immunity*
Pertussis	*Bordetella pertussis*	Airborne Direct contact	Man	7-10 days (not exceeding 21 days)	Early catarrhal stage to 3 weeks after onset of symptoms	Brain damage secondary infection malnutrition	Antibiotics	Prolonged
Tetanus	*Clostridium*	Broken skin	Man cattle spores found in soil	3-21 days	Not transmitted directly	Death	Sedatives muscle relaxants Antibiotics, Tetanus immunoglobulin	Clinical disease does not give immunity

Contd...

Contd...

Disease	*Causative agent*	*Mode of transmission*	*Reservoir*	*Incubation period*	*Communicability*	*Major complications*	*Specific treatment*	*Immunity*
Tuberculosis	*Mycobacterium tuberculosis bovis*	Air borne Raw Milk	Man cattle	4-12 weeks (may persist life time as latent infection)	Variable (as long as tubercle bacilli being discharged)	Progressive pulmonary disease Meningitis, Haematogenous (military)	Antimicrobials: Isoniazid and one or more of: Rifampicin, Streptomycin ethambutol or pyrazinamide	Variable

RECOMMENDED TEMPERATURE FOR STORAGE OF VACCINES

Sl No.	*Vaccine*	*Temperature in °C*	*Duration for which vaccine remains potent from the date of manufacture*	*Remarks*
1.	Oral Polio	<2°C	1 yr	Avoid repeated thawing. Keep on ice while using
		2°C - 8°C	3 Mo	-do-
2.	Measles	0°C - 8°C	2 yrs	–
3.	BCG	4°C - 8°C	2 yrs	Use within 3 hrs of dissolving
4.	DPT dual antigen	2°C - 8°C	2 yrs	Do not freeze
5.	DPT triple Antigen	2°C - 8°C	1 + yr	Do not freeze
6.	Typhoid	4°C - 10°C	1 + yr	Must not be freezed

Contd…

Contd...

Sl No.	*Vaccine*	*Tempe-rature in °C*	*Duration for which vaccine remains potent from the date of manufacture*	*Remarks*
7.	Tetanus Toxoid	2°C to 8°C	1 + yr	Do not freeze

- Vaccines should not be stocked for more than one month requirement
  - Vaccines are stored in ILR (Ice Lined Refrigerator)
  - ILR are top opening refrigerators
  - ILR has ice cubes/ice packs as ice lining.
  - The ice lines act as a buffer in case of power failure by preventing raise of temperature inside the refrigerator
  - There is no FREEZER COMPARTMENT in the ILR
  - The bottom of the ILR is the coldest place. DPT, DT, and TT should not be directly kept on the floor
  - Keep the dial thermometer inside the ILR to record the daily temperature (ILR also has an inbuilt thermometer).

THE DO'S AND DONT'S FOR USE OF ILR / FREEZER

Do's	*Dont's*
1. Keep the equipment in a cool room away from direct sunlight and at least 10 cms away from the wall. 2. Keep the equipment on a level ground 3. Fix the plug permanently to the socket 4. Use voltage stabilizer 5. Store the vaccines neatly with space between stacks for circulation of air 6. Keep the equipment locked and open if only when necessary 7. Defrost periodically. 8. Check the temperature twice a day and maintain a record 9. Take remedial action if the temperature is not maintained within the prescribed limit 10. Paste a notice outside the equipment that helps the user during a break down. • Whom to contact • Where to check for the blown fuse • Alternative place for vaccine storage	1. Do not keep drugs. 2. Do not open the door/top unless necessary 3. Do not keep food or drinking water in the refrigerator. 4. Do not keep anything for more than one month time in the refrigerator 5. Do not keep more than one month's requirements 6. Do not keep vaccines which are expired

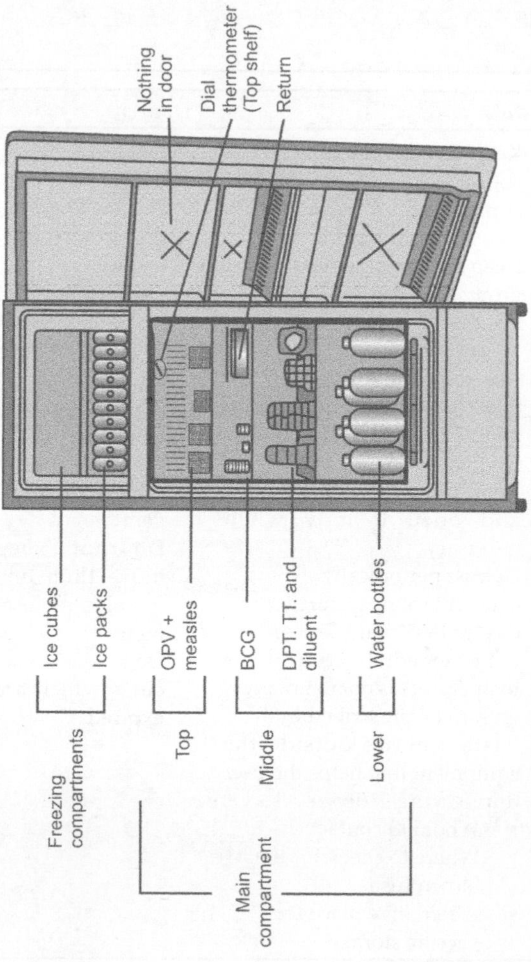

Refrigerator showing vaccines stored correctly in clinic setup

ILR FREEZER CHECKLIST FOR PREVENTIVE MAINTENANCE

Sl. No.	*Criteria*	*Yes*	*No*	*Sig*	*Remarks*
1.	The exterior is clean				
2.	It is firm on the floor				
3.	It is properly leveled				
4.	ILR is kept 10 cms away from the wall				
5.	The room is well ventilated				
6.	Lid is kept locked				
7.	Keys are kept at easily available place				
8.	Lid seals properly without gap				
9.	Lid seal is clean				
10.	Ice lining cubes/ice packs are in proper position				
11.	Ice lining cubes/ice packs are in proper level (no leak)				
12.	Thickness of frost formation is not more than 6 mm				
13.	Vaccines preserved in neat rows				
14.	There is space between rows for air circulation				
15.	DPT and TT vaccines are kept in the basket and not touching any cooling surface (for ILR only)				
16.	Reading of dial/stem thermometer				

Contd...

Contd...

Sl. No.	Criteria	Yes	No	Sig	Remarks
17.	Reading on the built in thermometer of the equipment				
18.	Temperature indicated is within specified range				
19.	Voltage stabilizer connected				
20.	Input voltage reading in volts				
21.	Output voltage reading in volts				
22.	Plug of voltage stabilizer fit properly (not loose)				
23.	Connections of equipment to voltage stabilizers proper and not loose				
24.	Compressor compartment and components inside are clean				
25.	Electrical connections are proper				
26.	No abnormal noise				
27.	Cooling fan works properly				
28.	Compressor and fan mounting bolts are tight				
29.	Pipe of components are not out of position not touching others				
30.	Temperature is recorded twice a day				

- For any negative answer take action

CHAPTER 8

Vitamin 'A' Deficiency

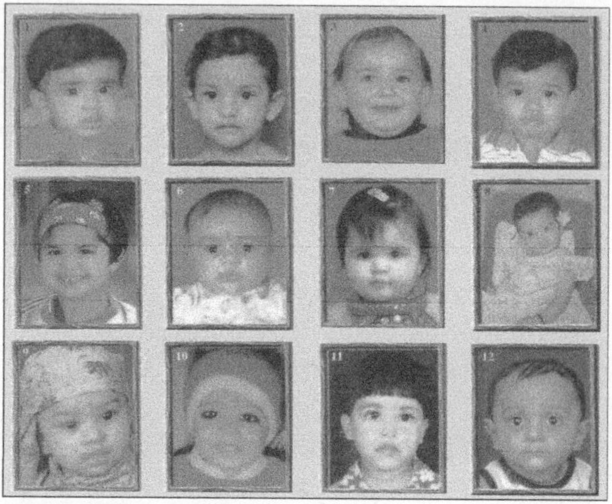

1. Vitamin 'A' deficiency is one of the common micronutrient deficiency in public health.
2. Vitamin 'A' deficiency leads to irreversible blindness in young children (widely prevalent between 6 mth and 3 yrs.)
3. Vitamin 'A' deficiency can be prevented.

SIGNS OF VITAMIN 'A' DEFICIENCIES

1. Night blindness.
2. Xerophthalmia – drying of conjunctiva and cornea. May progress into destruction of cornea, perforation and blindness.

3. Bitot's spots foamy cheesy material on conjunctiva.
4. The skin becomes dry and scaly. Hyperkeratosis may be found on shoulders, buttocks and extensor surfaces of extremities (Toad's skin).

PREVENTION OF VITAMIN 'A' DEFICIENCY

1. Dietary management : advice to include the following in diet: spinach, mango, papaya, milk, butter, cheese, egg, yolk, liver, animal fats, fish, liver oil
2. Vitamin A supplementation as follows:

Dose No.	*Age*	*Dose*	*Administered along with*
1.	On completion of 9 months	100000 IU	With measles vaccination
2.	15-18 months	200000 IU	With OPV, DPT booster
3	24 months	200000 IU	–
4	30 months	200000 IU	–
5	36 months	200000 IU	–

1. A total of 5 doses of Vit 'A' to be given at an interval of 6 months.
2. Promote vit 'A' rich foods (yellow veg, carrot, pumpkin, papaya, fish, yolk, etc.).

3. Educate the mother on the importance of giving colostrums and breast feeding.

TREATMENT OF VITAMIN A DEFICIENCY

1. Administer 200000 IU vit A solution following diagnosis.
2. Additional 200000 IU after 4 weeks.
3. Incase of infant the vit 'A' solution 100000 IU.
4. Children with eye lesions must be treated and referred to specialist.

ADDITIONAL POINTS

8

1. Vit 'A' concentrate solution is available in form of flavoured syrup in PHC.
2. Vit 'A' syrup is supplied in bottles with 2 ml spoon provided along with the bottle.
3. In case of measles out break, look for cases of vit A deficiency and act accordingly.

VIT 'A' PROPHYLAXIS SCHEDULE CHILDREN, AN, PN MOTHERS

Individual	*Oral dose of retinol palmitate*	*Timing*
Children < 12 months of age	55 mg (100000 IU)	Once every 4-6 months

Contd....

Contd....

Individual	*Oral dose of retinol palmitate*	*Timing*
Children > 12 Months of age	110 mg (200000 IU)	Once every 4-6 months
Newborn	27.5 mg (50000 IU)	At birth
Women of child bearing age	165 mg (300000 IU)	Within one month of giving birth
Pregnant and lactating women	2.75 mg (5000 IU) or	Every day
	11 mg (20000 IU)	Once every week

AN–Antenatal
PN–Postnatal

CHAPTER 9

Iron Deficiency Anaemia (In Children)

Causes: Anaemia is widely prevalent in India. The main cause includes recurrent diarrhea, worm infestation, insufficiency of iron in diet.

Diagnosis: Anaemia can be diagnosed by

1. Paleness of hands, lips, tongue, conjunctiva.
2. Estimation of Hb.
3. Stool examination for ova cyst.

Guidelines for the Diagnosis—Hb Estimation

Age group	*Hb (g/dl)*
6 months – 6 yrs	<11
6 yrs – 14 yrs	<12

TREATMENT

1. Administration of IFA (Iron and Folic Acid) tablets to 1-5 yrs of children with visible signs of anaemia
2. Administer IFA (small) daily for 100 days
3. Deworm (using Mebendazole 100 mg/twice daily) for 3 consecutive days before the IFA administration.

Prevention of Anaemia

1. Consume iron rich foods (egg, meat, green leafy vegetables – drumstick leaves, beetroot, jaggery, dates)
2. Prevent diarrhoeal infections

3. Administer Vit 'Complementary' along with iron for enhanced absorption
4. Treat helminthic infestation
5. Health education
6. General cleanliness of the mother, care taker and the child.

CHAPTER 10

Protein Energy Malnutrition (PEM)

PEM refers to a group of pathological conditions due to lack or deficit of proteins, calories in varying proportions among children under five years of age.

PREVALENCE OF PEM

Sl No.	Category – PEM	Prevalence
1.	PEM Mild	38% of preschool children
2.	PEM Moderate	44% of preschool children
3.	PEM Severe	9% of preschool children

- **PEM manifests itself by,**
  1. Growth failure
  2. Low body weight
  3. Nutritional hypoproteinemia.

CLASSIFICATION OF UNDERNUTRITION

Sl No.	Grade	Range – Comment with respect to RWA**
1	I	70-79% of RWA
2	II	60-69% of RWA
3	III	<60% of RWA
4	IV	50% of RWA

** RWA (Reference Weight for Age)

CLASSIFICATION OF PEM

- **PEM is classified on the basis of weight and presence of odema.**

Sl No.	*% of RWA*	*EDENA*	
		Present	**Absent**
1.	60-79.9	Kwashiorkor	Undernutrition
2.	<60	Marasmic kwashiorkor	Marasmus

DIFFERENCES / CLINICAL PICTURE OF KWASHIORKOR AND MARASMUS

Sl No.	*Criteria*	*Kwashiorkor*	*Marasmus*
1.	Prevalence	Less Common	Common than Kwashiorkor
2.	Incidence	Peak, 1-4 yrs	Peak incidence ½ -3 yrs
3.	Nutrition status	Case of imbalance	Case of balanced starvation
4.	Adaptation to food	Adaptation to low bulk	Failure of adaptation to low food bulk
5.	Emaciation	Emaciation masked by edema	Emaciation pronounced
6.	Edema/ ascitis	Edema (+), Ascitis (+)	Edema absent
7.	Skin, Hair changes	Present	No change

Contd...

Contd...

Sl No.	*Criteria*	*Kwashiorkor*	*Marasmus*
8.	Appetite	Lost	Good appetite
9.	Mental changes	Present	Absent
10.	Palpable liver	Some times palpable	Liver is never palpable
11.	Fatty in filteration of liver	Present	Normal liver
12.	Level of serum albumin	Reduced	Normal serum albumin level
13.	Prognosis	Poor ever with treatment	Prognosis is good

10

TREATMENT

Mild to Moderate case	*Severe PEM*
1. Give the child more foods	1. Needs admission in hospital
2. Increase the number of meals snacks to 5-6 times/day	2. Provide 200 kcal /kg of energy and 4 gm/kg of protein aggressively in kwashiorkor
3. Include given leafy vegetables in the child's diet	3. Treat accompanying nutritional deficiencies
4. Enrich the meal with the addition of a little oil, an egg or extra milk.	4. Detect complications like, dehydration, hypothermia, early and promptly treat
5. Ref to nutrition rehabilitation centre	5. Provide nutrition education to parents

CARDINAL FEATURES OF PEM

Principal Features of Severe PEM

Features	*Marasmus*	*Kwashiorkor*
CLINICAL	*ALWAYS PRESENT*	
Muscle wasting	Obvious	Sometimes hidden by oedema and fat
Fat wasting	Severe loss of subcutaneous fat	Fat often retained but not firm
Oedema	None	Present in lower legs, and usually in face and lower arms
Weight for height	Very low	Low but may be masked by oedema
Mental changes	Sometimes quiet and apathetic	Irritable, moaning, apathetic
CLINICAL	*SOMETIME PRESENT*	
Appetite	Usually good	Poor
Diarrhea	Often (current and past)	Often (current and past)
Skin changes	Usually none	Diffuse pigmentation, sometimes flaky paint dermatosis
Hair changes	Seldom	Sparse, Silky, Easily pluckable

Contd...

Contd...

Hepatic enlargement	None	Sometimes, due to accumulation of fat
BIOCHEMICAL		
Serum albumin	Normal or slightly decreased	Low (<3 g / 100 ml blood)
Urinary urea per g creatinine	Normal or decreased	Low
Hydroxy-proline/ creatinine ratio	Low	Low
Plasma/amino acid ratio	Normal	Elevated

Reproduced from Text book of Social and Preventive Medicine K. Park

PREVENTION OF PEM

1. Education and advise on home made high protein mixture

Home Made Protein Mixture

Sl No.	*Ingredient*	*Qty*
1	Ragi	250 gms
2	Wheat / Rice	250 gms
3	Green gram	250 gms
4	Ground nuts	100 gms
5	Til (sesame)	50 gms
6	Sugar / jaggery	300 gms

- The ingredients are separately fried
- Then the ingredients are mixed together
- Add sugar/jaggery and whole ground
- The resulting powder is stored in a tin with tight lid
- 60 gms is mixed with a little water to form porridge and fed to the children two times a day
- The powder can also be mixed with little ghee and made into ladoos
- Administer 2 ladoos a day

2. Educate the mothers on the importance of breast feeding
3. Educate the mother on the importance of growth monitoring
4. Advice nutritional supplementation.

CHAPTER 11

Diarrhoea Management

WHAT IS DIARRHOEA?

1. Passage of frequent formed stools.
2. Passage of pasty stools in breast fed infants.
3. Passage of stools during or immediately following feeds due to gastrocolic reflex.
4. Transitional stools on the third to seventh day of life.

ASSESSMENT OF DEHYDRATION

Sl No.		*No Dehydration*	*Dehydration*	*Severe Dehydration*
1.	Look	Well alert	Restless irritable	Lethargic or unconscious or flabby
2.	Thirst	Not thirsty drinks normally	Thirsty drinks eagerly	Drinks poorly or not able to drink
3.	Skin pinch	Goes back quickly	Goes back slowly	Goes back very slowly
4.	Mouth and tongue	Moist	Dry	Very dry
5.	Eyes	Normal	Sunken	Very sunken

ORS AND ITS CONTENTS

The composition of WHO ORS (Net wt = 27.9 gms)

Sl No.	*Ingredients*	*Wt (gms)*	*In mEq/Lt*
1.	Sodium chloride IP	3.5	90 mEq/Lt
2	Potassium chloride IP	1.5	20 mEq/Lt
3.	Sodium citrate IP	2.9	30 mEq/Lt
4.	Glucose Anhydrous IP	20	110 mmol/Lt

MANAGEMENT OF CHILD WITH DIARRHOEA AT HOME FLUID REPLACEMENT

Age	*Qty to be Administered*
<6 months	After each liquid stool, ¼ glass (50 ml)
6 months – 2 yrs	¼ - ½ glass (50-100 ml)
2-5 yrs	½ - 1 glass (100 – 200 ml)

MANAGEMENT OF CHILD WITH DIARRHOEA WITH NO DEHYDRATION

1. Administer HAF (Home Available Fluids)/ ORS as long as diarrhoea lasts.

2. Continue breast feeding (appropriate for the age). If the child is on exclusive breast feed, breast feed is enough to prevent dehydration
3. Food normally taken should be continued.

GUIDELINES FOR REHYDRATION THERAPY

Age	*<4 Mo.*	*4-11 Mo*	*12-23 Mo*	*2-4 yrs*	*5-14 yrs*
Wt in kgs	<5 kg	5-8	8-11	11-16	16-39
ORS (ml)	200-400	400-600	600-800	800-1200	1200-2200
Measure glass	1-2	2-3	3-4	4-6	6-11

- Advise to continue BF along with ORS (Breast feeding)

POINTS FOR HEALTH EDUCATION TO THE MOTHER

1. Administer one tea spoon for every 1-2 min.
2. To an older child, give frequent–sips from a cup/glass.
3. If the child vomits, wait for 10 min, then start giving slowly.
4. If ORS packets are exhausted, continue HAF
5. If the child develops puffiness of the eyelids, discontinue ORS.
   (Administer plain water/breast milk).

11

INDICATIONS TO DISCONTINUE ORAL REHYDRATION

Discontinue ORS, if the child,

1. Vomits persistently.
2. Not able to take fluids orally.
3. Becomes more dehydrated.
4. Fails to pass urine for 8 hrs.
5. Develops complications, like abdominal distension, drowsiness or conclusions.

Prevention of Diarrhoea

1. Educate the mother about the causes of diarrhoea.
2. Advocate exclusive breast feeding upto 6 months of age.
3. Measles vaccination at 9-12 months of age.
4. Avoid contamination of food.
5. Wash hands before and after eating.
6. Use safe drinking water.
7. Use latrine for defecation.
8. Advice Vit 'A' rich diet.

CHAPTER 12

Acute Respiratory Infections (ARI)

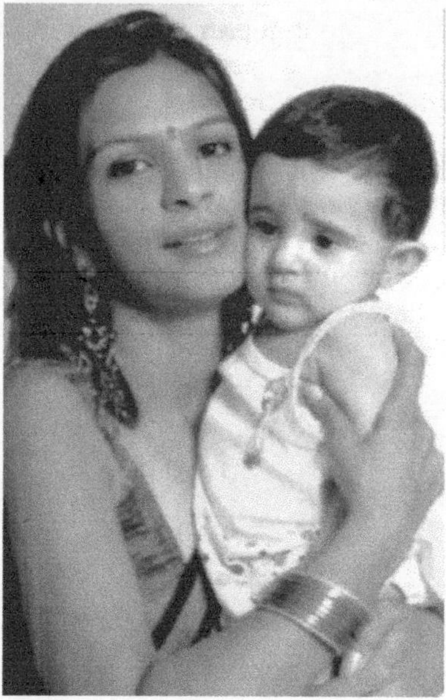

INTRODUCTION

A child in an urban area suffers from 5-9 episodes of ARI, and 1-3 episodes in rural area.

ARI

Refers to infection of respiratory tract less than 30 days duration, excluding otitis media less than 14 days.

CLASSIFICATION

1. Upper Respiratory Tract Infections (URI)
2. Lower Respiratory Tract Infections (LRI)

URI includes common cold, pharyngitis, laryngitis, tracheitis, epiglotitis, and otits media.

LRI includes bronchitis, bronchiolitis and pneumonias.

Diagnosis

1. History taking
2. Assessment of respiratory rate (Breathing Pattern).
3. Look for signs of chest indrawing.

MANAGEMENT

Sl No.	*Condition*	*Intervention*	*Place of Treatment*
1.	**No Pneumonia** • Cough (+) • No fast breathing • No chest indrawing	Home remedies	Home

Contd...

Contd...

Sl No.	*Condition*	*Intervention*	*Place of Treatment*
2.	**Pneumonia** • Cough (+) (+) • Fast Breathing (+)(+) **Breathing rate and age** • 2 Mo – 12 Mo: 50/min or > • 12 Mo – 60 Mo : 40/min or > • No chest indrawing	Co-Trimaxazole tablet	• Home or • Health centre
3.	**Severe Pneumonia** • Fast breathing <2Mo : RR-60/min with or without chest indrawing • 2 Mo - 12 Mo : RR-50/min or more • 12 Mo - 60 Mo : RR 40/min or more • Chest indrawing inability to drink • Lethargic • Excessive drowsiness • Stridor in a calm child • Cyanosis • Convulsions • S/S severe malnutrition • Hypothermia	Antibiotics Oxygen	Hospital/ Secondary or tertiary care centre

GUIDELINES FOR MANAGEMENT OF A CASE OF PNEUMONIA

(Tab Septran)/Co-Trimaxazole Dosage

Age/Wt.	*Pediatric Tablet Sulfamethoxazole 100 mgm and Trimethoprim*	*Pediatric Syrup Each tea spoon (5 ml) Sulfamethoxazole 200 mg and Trimethoprim*
<2 Mo. Wt: 3.5 kg	1 tab/twice a day	½ tsp (2.5 ml)/twice a day
22 Mo. Wt: 6-9 kg	2 tab/twice a day	1 tsp (5 ml)/twice a day
1-5 Yrs Wt: 10-19 kg	3 tab/twice a day	1 and ½ tsp (7.5 ml)/ twice a day

Note:

1. Do not administer tab septran to premature babies/with neonatal Jaundice.
2. The tablets are to be crushed and mixed with water and administered using a spoon.

TREATMENT OF PNEUMONIA USING ANTIBIOTICS

Antibiotics	*Dosage*	*Frequency*		*Route*
		Age <7 days	*7 days – 2 Mo*	
Inj Benzyl (or) penicillin	5000 IU kg/dose	12 hrly	6 hrly	IV/IM

Contd...

Contd...

Antibiotics	*Dosage*	*Frequency*		*Route*
		Age <7 days	*7 days – 2 Mo*	
Inj Ampicillin and	50 mg kg/dose	12 hrly	8 hrly	IV/IM
Inj Gentamycin	2.5 mg/ kg/dose	12 hrly	8 hrly	IV/IM

12

MANAGEMENT OF ARI (MILD – MODERATE USING HOME REMEDIES)

1. Extract of Tulsi leaves (Boilded and extracted) could be administered with honey (1 tsp Tulsi extract + 1 tsp honey) thrice a day.
2. Lukewarm milk with a pinch of turmeric powder could be administered.
3. One pinch of pepper powder (black pepper) can be administered once/twice a day depending on the age of the child along with honey.

HEALTH EDUCATION TO THE MOTHER

Advise the mothers on the following:

1. The method and relevant information on the administration of antibiotics.
2. To continue adequate feeding in small quantity in frequent intervals.

3. On s/s of improvement of the child to the treatment.
4. Warning signs are taught so that the mother can appropriately decide about reporting to the referral centre.

   The warning signs are as follows :
   - Dyspnoea or rapid breathing
   - Chest indrawing
   - Refusal of feeds
   - Eating and drinking poorly
   - Excessive sleeping/drowsiness
   - Convulsions
   - Cyanosis.

HOME MANAGEMENT FOR COMMON COLD, COUGH AND FEVER WITHOUT S/S PNEUMONIA

Advise the mother to the following to:

1. Continue feeding as before
2. Advise feed in small frequent intervals
3. Encourage to give more fluids orally
4. Administer antipyretics if there is raise of temperature
5. Clean the nose with normal saline drops and gently remove the crusts
6. Give honey, ginger (tulsi, for children above 2 months)

7. Educate the mother to monitor the childs progress and to identify warning signs at the earliest.

PREVENTION OF ARI

1. Exclusively breast feed the child for 6 months
2. Avoid exposure to dusty and smoky environment
3. Administer DPT, BCG, Measles and Polio vaccinations as per the immunization schedule
4. Administer Vit 'A' Prophylaxis 9 Mo – 6 yrs (100000 IU/200000 IU at 6 months intervals)
5. Promote and maintain adequate nutrition
6. Advice Vit 'A' rich diet.

CHAPTER 13

Antenatal Care

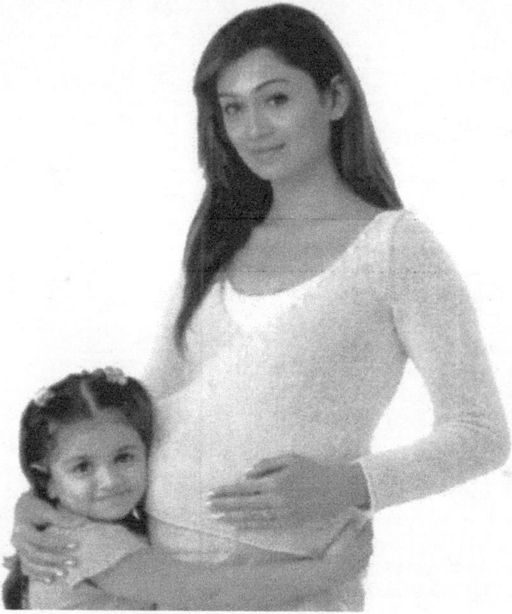

AIMS AND OBJECTIVES OF MCH/RCH SERVICES

- To give expert advice to the couples to plan their families
- Provide health supervision for AN mothers
- To detect "High Risk" cases and provide special attention
- To foresee complications and prevent them

- To give skilled assistance at the time of child birth and during puerperium
- To supervise trained dais
- To give newborn and child health supervision
- To impart useful knowledge on desirable health practices to be adopted during provision of MCH care.

ANTENATAL CARE / AN CARE

Aims of Antenatal Care

- To promote and maintain good mental and physical health during pregnancy
- To monitor the progress of pregnancy
- To detect and treat medical and obstetrical condition
- To ensure safe delivery and mature and healthy infant
- To prepare the women for delivery, breast feeding and subsequent care of the child
- To encourage concept of having regular AN care.

Importance of Antenatal Care

- To confirm pregnancy and assess the period of gestation
- To prevent maternal and neonatal tetanus

- To facilitate health education regarding diet, rest, avoidance of unnecessary travel and preparation for delivery.

Components of AN Care

- Identification of pregnant women and importance of early registration
- Diagnosis of pregnancy
- Clinical assessment
- Nutrition
- Management of minor ailments
- Risk assessment and appropriate management
- Complication and management
- Complication of late pregnancy
- Management of medical disorders during pregnancy
- Screening for congenital malformations during pregnancy
- Management of Anaemia during pregnancy.

IDENTIFICATION REGISTRATION—12 WKS

Early Identification Helps

- Assessing the health status of the mother
- Obtain baseline information of the mother
- Screen for factors, referral to FRU
- Recall LMP easily
- Do MTP if required (<10 wks)

- Counsel on hygiene, diet, rest
- Build up rapport with pregnant women.

Within 20 WKS

- Screen and treat anaemia
- Initiate prophylaxis
- Screen risk factors and medical conditions
- Develop individualized birth plan
- Immunize with tetanus toxoid
- Investigate – Hb, blood group, typing, urine examination, VDRL.

28–32 WKS

Aimed at the following; Detect

- PIH
- Multiple gestation
- Anaemia
- Develop individualized birth plan
- Give TT
- Assess IUGR
- Repeat Hb estimation.

36 WKS – Assess

Detect the following

- PIH
- Identify fetal and presentation
- Rule out CPD in primi gravida.

Diagnosis of Pregnancy

Women may report with symptoms of
- Cessation of menstruation
- Nausea with or without vomiting
- Disturbance in micturation
- Fatigue
- Perception of foetal movements.

O/E..............Find

- Breast enlargement
- Changes in skin colour of areola
- Discoloration of vaginal mucosa
- Enlargement of abdomen
- Softening of cervix and uterus
- Uterine enlargement
- Internal and external ballottement
- Ability to discern fetal parts.

13

Clinically

- Perception of fetal movements by the examiner
- Detection of fetal heart sounds at 20 wks
- Detection of HCG in urine
- Detection of fetus and placenta on USG.

Clinical Assessment : Assess

- Age
- Duration of marriage

- The order of pregnancy
- Number of living children
- A general history – Date, LMP
- Last child birth
- Last abortion
- Problems during previous pregnancy.

Problems During Previous Pregnancy

- Abortion or premature birth
- Eclampsia/pre-eclampsia
- APH
- Malaria, anaemia, UTI
- Complicated delivery, PROM (Premature rupture of membranes)
- Sepsis
- Operations
- Still birth, neonatal death
- Induced labour
- Baby weight at birth, sex, alive well.

History of Systemic Illness: H/O

- Heart disease
- DM
- TB
- HT
- UTI
- Malaria
- Thyroid diseases.

Family History

- Twins
- Congenitally malformed baby.

Complication during Present Pregnany

- Breathlessness
- Excessive tiredness
- Palpitation
- Puffiness of face
- Tightening of bangles
- Headache, blurring of vision
- Bleeding, Leaking PV
- Pain abdomen, fever, presence of fetal movements.

Physical Examination

- Height
- Weight
- BP, Hb, grouping, typing U/S, U/A
- Pallor
- Oedema
- Breast examination
- Respiratory rate
- CVS – prominent neck vein.

Fundal height in pregnancy

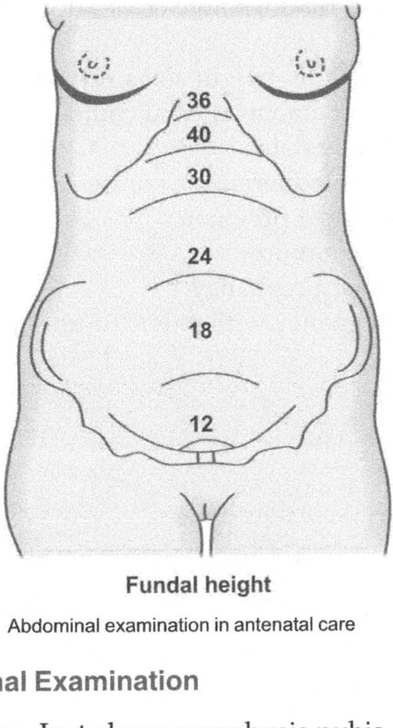

Fundal height

Abdominal examination in antenatal care

Abdominal Examination

- 16 wks – Just above symphysis pubis
- 20 wks – Midway between symphysis pubis and umbilicus
- 24 wks – At the level of umbilicus upper two-third of distance between umbilicus and xiphisternum

- 28 wks –
- 40 wks – fundal height comes down but flanks are full
- If the fundal height does not correlate with period of amenorrhea, it could be due to:
  - Wrong dates
  - Full bladder
  - Multiple pregnancy
  - Hydramnios
  - Molar pregnancy
  - Pregnancy with pelvic tumor.

If Less

- Wrong dates
- IUGR
- Missed abortion
- IUD
- Molar pregnancy
- Transverse lie.

Advice During a Visit

- Iron and folic acid supplementation
- TT injections (2), 4-6 wks apart, if the previous child birth was within 3 yrs – 1 dose TT
- To bring AN card during every visit
- Pregnant women may continue her usual activities throughout her pregnancy if not tired

- Hard and strenuous work should be avoided
- Should take bath daily
- Should sleep for 8-10 hrs at night and 2 hrs during day
- Clean loose cotton cloth should be worn
- Retracted nipples should be corrected during the last 6 wks
- Coitus should be avoided during 1st and last trimester
- Travel by vehicles having jerks is to be avoided
- AN mothers and the attender to be told regarding minor ailments and waring signs and do's and don't's.

Risk Assessment and Management

Obstetric Factor

- Gravity – primigravida/grand multipara
- Age - > 35 yrs below 19 yrs
- Height - < 145 cm (pre pregnancy wt less or over weight 20% as per height weight standard)
- Multipara with BOH – loss of previous baby, caesarian section, HT, recurrent premature labour, abortion, IU fetal death, III stage abnormalities, congenital malformations, neonatal deaths
- Cases of disproportion — pelvic contraction, pelvic tumor primigravida with non-engaged head at/near term

- Malpresentations/multiple pregnancy.
- Obstetric complications—haemorrhage, threatened abortion, APH, PIH
- High risk fetus – premature labour, IUGR, RH incompatibility, postmaturity
- Infertility – conceived after treatment for infertility.

MEDICAL FACTORS

Refer to FRU in following Situation:

- BOH—repeated abortion (BOH – Bad Obstetrical History)
- Bleeding during pregnancy
- PIH/Eclampsia
- Abnormal presentations
- Multiple pregnancy/over distended uterus
- Grand multipara
- Previous history of operative surgery
- Floating head in primigravida at 38 wks and later
- Preterm labour.

NUTRITION

Dietary Advice during Pregnancy

- Advice a diet that is nutritious easily digestable, rich in protein, minerals and vitamins

consisting of normal foods plus.....at least
- Half litre milk/day
- One egg
- Plenty of green leafy vegetables
- Fruits
- Fiber rich diet

- Advice extra calories for maternal health and to meet the needs of the growing foetus
- Advice diet keeping in mind the socio-economic condition.

Management of Minor Ailments

1. Vomiting in Pregnancy
    - Wanes off at 12-14 wks
    - Advice small frequent foods
    - Avoid greasy foods
    - Include plenty of green leafy vegetables
    - Advice plenty of fluids
    - Encourage dry foods in the morning.
2. Heart Burn and Nausea
    - Avoid spicy, rich foods
    - Take cold milk and bland diet
    - If severe administer antacids
3. Frequency of Micturation
   Experienced more frequently upto 10-12 wks and is mostly self limiting
4. Constipation
    - Encourage increased fiber intake

5. Others
   - Premature rupture of membrane labour pain does not start within 6 hrs
   - Very big or very small baby
   - Hyperemesis gravidarum not responding to treatment
   - Heart diseases in pregnancy
   - Jaundice in pregnancy.
6. Complications of Early Pregnancy
   - Hyperemesis gravidaram
   - Retroverted gravid uterus with retention of urine
   - Vaginal bleeding during pregnancy.

PREVENTION OF ANAEMIA

Causes

- Iron deficiency
- Folic acid deficiency
- Iron and folic acid deficiency
- Nutritional

Types of Anaemia

- Hyper chromic microcytic anaemia
- Macrocytic anaemia
- Dimorphic anaemia
- Normocytic normochromic anaemia

Investigations

- Hb investigation
- Stool for cyst
- Urine analysis, UTI
- Hb electrophorosis

Treatment

- Mild - moderate – oral Fe+ and Folic Acid
- Diet rich in protein and iron
- Vit C supplementation
- Treatment of UTI
- Oral iron
- Supplementation of vitamins
- Referral to FRU

Calculation of Iron Requirement

For parenteral Iron supplementation:

Wt in pounds × deficit of Hb. × 3 + 300 mg

Oral

1. Prophylactic – IFA Large–1/day Supplementation
2. Therapeutic – IFA Large – 2/day. Complications of Anaemia during Pregnancy
   - Pre term labour
   - Prone to infections

- CCF, APH, PPH, Maternal mortality
- IUGR, Prematurity, IUD

Complication in Late Pregnancy include

- IUD Pre-eclampsia
- Eclampsia
- PROM
- IUGR
- CCF–Congestive cardiac failure
- APH–Ante partum hemorrhage
- PPH–Post partum hemorrhage
- IUGR–Intra uterine growth retardation
- IUD–Intra uterine death
- PROM–Premature rupture of membranes

Pre-eclampsia

Definition

Is development of hypertension with or without proteinuria with edema, induced by pregnancy, after 20 wks of pregnancy.

Diagnosis

- BP-140/90 mmHg
- Or sudden/excessive wt gain
  Weight gain > 1 kg/wk or 3 kg/month

Management

- BED REST-Lt lateral position
- Examination twice a week
- Control of BP – Nifidipine 10 mg (oral) or sublingually
- ....Sedation – Inj Largectil 50 mg IM
- ....Inj Diazepam 100 mg IM
- Refer to FRU

ECLAMPSIA

Hypertension, Proteinuria, oedema, convulsions charecterize eclampsia

Management

Refer to FRU
Before referal – Administer Diazepam 10 Mg IM, Nifedipine 10 mg Sublingually

During Transportation

- Women must lie on sides and head turned
- Put soft gags between teeth
- Monitor BP every 20 min
- Establish IV line with splint
- Give oxygen
- Start antibiotics
- Do continuous catheterization.

PROM

Spontaneous rupture of membranes anytime during pregnancy beyond 28 wks, before the labour is termed as premature rupture of membranes.

Confirmation of Diagnosis

Speculum examination
PH detection (7-7.5 – liquor amni)
Fern test

Treatment

- Minimal vaginal examination
- Start antibiotics (amoxy 500 mg 6 hrly)
- Bed rest
- Refer to FRU
- Conduct delivery

IUGR IS A CONDITION

When the birth weight is below 10% of the average for gestational age.

Management

- Take adequate bed rest
- Avoid smoking and alcohol
- Correct malnutrition
- Refer to FRU.

Medical Disorders During Pregnancy

- Pregnancy with heart disease
- Pregnancy with diabetes
- Pregnancy with UTI
- Pregnancy with jaundice
- Pregnancy with TB
- Pregnancy with malaria

SCREENING FOR CONGENITAL MALFORMATIONS HIGH RISK FACTORS

- Hydramnios
- Severe IUGR
- Abnormal presentation
- Elderly mother
- History of drug intake
- Uncontrolled DM
- Hypothyroidism – of the mother
- H/O mentally retarded off springs in the family

Prevention

- Administration of folic acid 5 mg daily – months before conception
- Prevention of all kinds of infection
- Early diagnosis of malformation and termination
- Avoidance of medication (without physician's prescription).

CHAPTER 14

Intranatal Care

EUTOCIA

Normal labour or eutocia is the process of expulsion per vaginum of a mature live foetus presented by vertex followed by placenta and membranes spontaneously without any complication of delay.

STAGES OF LABOUR

First Stage

The first stage starts from the onset of labour pains till full dilation of cervix; usually 12 hrs in primigravida and 6 hrs in multipara.

Second Stage

From dilation of cervix to expulsion of foetus, it lasts 2 hrs in nullipara and 1 hr in multipara.

Third Stage

From expulsion of foetus till the delivery of placenta. Third stage of labour lasts for 5 to 10 min it should not exceed 30 min.

SIGNS OF TRUE LABOUR

Diagnose Labour by the Following Signs

- Painful uterine cantractions, at regular intervals, progressively increasing in duration and intensity

- Progressive cervical dilation and effacement
- Formation of bag of waters
- Presence of show.

MANAGEMENT OF FIRST STAGE OF LABOUR

Ensure

- The bowel is emptied by enema
- The women is given clean gown to wear and to be ambulant
- Posture – Ambulant, lying flat on her back may give supine hypotension
- Nutrition – Clear fluids are given to prevent dehydration, solid foods are avoided to prevent any anesthetic complication if surgery is required
- Bladder – She passes frequently as full bladder may delay the progress of labour.

MONITORING THE FIRST STAGE OF LABOUR AND MAINTENANCE OF PARTOGRAM

- Partograph is a tool to monitor the progress and management of labour
- Partograph is used to record all observations made on a woman in labour
- Its central feature is a graph where dilation of the cervix assessed by vaginal examination is plotted

- By noting the rate at which the cervix dilates, one can assess the normalcy of labour, therefore, partograph is a powerful tool.

Advantages of Partograph

- Partograph helps to prevent prolonged and obstructed labour
- It is a clear way of recording all observations on one chart
- Helps in detecting abnormalities
- It is a potent tool to manage labour.

Usage of Partograph

Observe and record in the following sequence:
- Cervical dilation
- Descent of head
- Uterine contraction
- Duration show by differential shading
- The foetal condition
- The maternal condition.

Monitor Foetal Condition

- Observing the foetal heart rate is safe and reliable clinical way of knowing the wellbeing of the foetus.
  - A rate >160 beats/min (tachycardia), <120/min (bradycardia) may indicate foetal distress.

- A heart beat <100 or lower indicates very severe distress and action should be taken at once.

Monitoring Maternal Condition

Monitor the following:

- Pulse – half hourly
- Blood pressure 4 hourly and frequently as indicated
- Temperature – 4 hourly and frequently as indicated
- Urine volume – encourage women to pass 2-4 hourly and maintain I/O chart
- Drugs and IV fluid – chart these in appropriate columns
- Oxytocin regime.

IDENTIFICATION OF MANAGEMENT OF FOETAL AND MATERNAL DISTRESS

Evidence of Foetal Distress

- Persistence of tachycardia >160/min
- Persistence of bradycardia <120/min
- Irregularity of foetal heart sound
- Excessive foetal movements
- Passage of meconium per vaginum in cephalic presentation

If any of the signs do not improve despite management labour has to be terminated either by LSCS in first stage or by Instrumental delivery — refer to FRU.

Management

- Oxygen inhalation
- To lie in left position
- Inj Ringer Lactate
- Shift to FRU.

Evidences of Maternal Distress

The following are the signs of Maternal Distress:

- Increased pulse rate >100/min
- Looks exhausted
- Rise of temp > 104°F
- Dehydrated tongue
- Appearance of protein and ketones in urine (ketostix, Rothera test).

Management

- Start IV 5% dextrose, followed by RL infusion
- Reassess the progress of labour
- Assess the type of uterine contraction
- Assess the foetal condition
- Manage accordingly.

MANAGEMENT OF II STAGE OF LABOUR

Diagnosis of II Stage

- Mother vomits or reports that she feels a need to defecate
- Membranes spontaneously rupture
- Mother has intense urge to bear down during contraction
- PV – cervix is no longer palpable (i.e.) fully dilated.

Conduct of Delivery

Shift the mother to delivery room when the foetal head is seen at vulva in between contraction

- Monitor FHR every 5 min
- Bring the mother to the edge of the table preferably in dorsal or semirecumbent position
- Wash perineal area with an antiseptic solution and use sterile drapers
- When the head is crowning the perineum make a decision as to the requirement of Episiotomy (Episiotomy are routinely given to all the mothers).

Episiotomy : Infiltration

Give local infiltration with 1% xylocaine along the line of planned episiotomy cut which is usually a mediolateral one.

- If the episiotomy is made at the right time, almost with the next contraction and patients bearing down effort, the head will deliver
- Apply countertraction anteriorly to the vertex with one hand while a towel or pad in the other hand supports the perineum to enable a controlled delivery of the head rather than a sudden pop out
- Once the head is delivered, palpate the fetal neck to see for loop of cord wrapped around it, if the loop is loose slip it over the head posteriorly but if it is tight it is cut between two clamps
- Clear the baby's mouth and oropharynx with mucous sucker before the body delivers. Deliver the shoulders by depressing the head posteriorly so that the lateral flexion of the body occurs. The rest of the body automatically follows
- At the delivery of the anterior shoulder give IV methergine 0.2 mg unless there is contraindication. Methergine is contraindicated in hypertensive conditions
- Cut the cord between clamps and hand ever the baby to paediatrician
- Note the time of the birth of the baby
- Give the baby to the mother and let the baby start sucking at the breast.

MANAGEMENT OF III STAGE OF LABOUR

- Place the left hand on lower abdomen to detect the contraction of uterus
- Following the delivery uterus is just below the umbilicus.

Signs of Placental Separation

- Uterus becomes hard and globular
- Uterus raises just below umbilicus
- Note for extra vulval lengthening of the umbilical cord
- A gush of blood frequently appears
- On pushing the uterine up in the abdomen the cord does not recede back
- Placenta is delivered by controlled cord traction and concentration of the uterine corpus
- Cord traction should be avoided before the placenta is separated
- If methergine is not given, 0.2 mg IM should be given after the delivery of the placenta
- Inspect the placenta for completeness. Feel the hard retracted uterus and if the vaginal bleeding is not excessive, proceed to inspect the vagina for evidence of any laceration or tears
- Repair of the tears and Episitomy is done on similar lines.

Episiotomy (Perineotomy)

Perineotomy is an incision into the perineum to enlarge the space at the outlet, thereby facilitating the birth of the child.

Indications for Episiotomy

- To preserve the integrity of the pelvic floor
- To prevent uncontrolled perineal tear
- To prevent foetal head in preterm babies, large babies, abnormal positions and in breech presentations.

Perineal Tears

Many women suffer from tears of perineum. The following are the types:

First degree tear: The vaginal mucosa, superficial tissues of perineum are involved but does not injure muscular tissue.

Second degree tear: The perineal muscles are torn.

Third degree tear: The tear extends through the perineal body, muscles and the anal splinter and occasionally anterior rectal wall.

HEALING OF THE PERINEUM

Ensure

- General hygiene
- Low residue diet for three days

- Laxatives to make stool soft
- Avoid enema
- Ambulate the mother
- Encourage fluid intake.

EQUIPMENTS OF NORMAL DELIVERY—LABOUR ROOM

- Catheters – Simple catheter and self retaining catheters
- Enema apparatus
- Sponge holding forceps
- Scissors
- Dissecting forceps
- Needle – Round bodied, cutting
- Needle holder
- Artery forceps
- Sutures - chronic catgut. No-1 on round body and cutting needle
- Obstetrics forceps
- Kidney trays
- Bowls
- Rubber sheets
- Thermometer
- BP apparatus
- Episiotomy tray
- Episiotomy scissors
- Small curved artery forceps

- For local infiltration–10 ml syringe hypodermic needle, antiseptic solution, sterile drapes and cotton swabs
- Gowns and masks
- Sterilized rubber gloves.

IDENTIFICATION OF ABNORMAL PROGRESS OF LABOUR

Is characterized by
- Prolonged latent phase
- Abnormalities of the descent.

Malpresentations

- Unanticipated breech in the II stage
- Face presentation
- Cord relapse and cord presentation
- Undiagnosed twins.

OBSTRUCTED LABOUR AND THREATENING RUPTURE

Primary Management

- Stop syntocinon if started
- Oxygen inhalation/left lateral position
- Sedation
- Catheterization of the bladder
- IV dextrose saline to be given

- Antibiotics to be started
- Ref to FRU
- Terminate labour and prevent rupture of UT with a note of treatment given with blood donors.

POSTPARTUM HAEMORRHAGE

It is the loss of blood in excess of 500 ml with detrimental effect on the mother's condition.

Types

- Primary haemorrhage
- Secondary haemorrhage

PRIMARY HAEMORRHAGE

The term is used when bleeding occurs within 24 hours following the birth of the baby.

Types (Based on Causes)

- Atonic haemorrhage
- Traumatic haemorrhage

Atonic

When the uterus fails to contract and retract effectively to stop bleeding, it is termed as atonic uterine haemorrhage. The predisposing factors are:

- Grand multipara
- Over distension of uterus
- Malnutrition and anaemia
- APH
- Prolonged labour
- Oxytocin use
- Malformation of uterus
- Uterine fibroid
- Mis-managed third stage of labour.

Traumatic Uterine Bleeding

- Episiotomy, extension of episiotomy
- Vaginal tear
- Cervical tear
- Vulval tear (Paraurethral tears)
- Cervical tears, extending into uterus.

Mixed PPH

Combination of Atonic and Traumatic and Blood Coagulopathies

- Abruptio placenta
- Pre-eclampsia and Eclampsia
- IUD
- Jaundice in pregnancy
- Thrombocytopenic purpura.

Clinical Features

- Combined features, vaginal bleeding, copious blood, or slow trickle
- Concealed hematomas (concealed haemorrhage)
- Effect depends on pre-delivery haemoglobin and blood loss
- Rapid pulse and fall in BP
- The uterus may be flabby (atonic)
- Well contracted in case of traumatic.

Management

- Inj Ergometrine 0.25 mg/methergine 0.2 mg IV
- Start IV with RL, add 20 units syntocinon
- Oxygen mask if hypoxia develops
- Catheterize if bladder is full
- Give bimanual uterine massage if uterus in atonic
- Explore genital tract for tear
- Repair the tear immediately.

Prevention of PPH (Primary)

- Improve Hb atenatally
- Screen high risk patients and refer to FRU
- Avoid kneading or fiddling of the uterus and pulling of the crod in III stage

- Examine placenta and membranes. Detect missing cotyledons
- In case of induced labour continue syntocinon infusion for at least one hour after delivery
- Administer ergometrine with the delivery of anterior shoulder
- Explore vagina and uterus for trauma
- Observe the mother for 2 hrs before shifting
- Put the child to breast soon after delivery.

SECONDARY POSTPARTUM HAEMORRHAGE

Occurs after 24 hrs or within 42 days of the delivery.

Causes

- Retained bits of placenta
- Infection
- Inversion of uterus
- Placental polyp.

Management

May need referral to FRU if blood loss is excessive for exploration under anaesthesia.

- Inj methergine 0.2 mg IM, 8 hourly for 24 hrs followed by T. Methergine, one tablet twice a day – 3 days
  - Antibiotics
  - Bed rest
  - Definitive treatment of the cause.

Shock

Shock is state of collapse of blood circulation resulting in critical reduction of tissue perfusion.

Types

- Haemorrhagic shock
- Non-haemorrhagic shock

Haemorrhagic Shock

Bleeding is the commonest cause of haemorrhagic shock. It causes hypovolaemia.

Non-haemorrhagic Shock

Postpartum collapse is due to:
- Inversion of uterus
- Retained placenta without bleeding
- Prolonged labour – acidosis, infection
- Traumatic operative delivery
- Amniotic fluid embolism and Hypofibrinogenemia
- Pulmonary embolism.

Clinical Features

Clinically mother may have sweating, feeling of restlessness, tachycardia, low volume pulse, low BP, subnormal temperature and oliguria.

Management

- Inj morphine sulphate 15 mg IM to relieve pain
- Continuous oxygen inhalation
- Ensure patent airway
- Raise the foot end of the patient
- Fluid therapy rapid infusion of glucose saline to restore the blood volume
- Steroid hormones, Inj hydrocortisone 500 - 1000 mg is useful in all kinds of shock
- Monitor vital signs for improvement
- Refer to FRU for further management.

Pulmonary Embolism

Is characterized by

- Sudden collapse
- Acute chest pain
- Air hunger
- Pleural pain
- Hemoptysis.

O/E Exhibits

- Cyanosis
- Increased RR
- Distension of Jugular vein
- Pleural rub
- Death usually occurs within short time from shock.

Management

- Propped up position
- Oxygen inhalation
- Sedation
- Lasix 40 mg IV
- Maintenance of IV line

CHAPTER 15

Postnatal Care

15

INTRODUCTION

Postnatal period (or) Puerperium begins after the third stage of labour till the first 6 weeks following the delivery.

POSTNATAL VISIT

Advice the mother as follows:

- At least two postnatal visits are must
- First visit – within 10 days of delivery
- Second visit – 6 weeks of delivery.

Aims of First Visit

- Obtain history on
  - Delivery
  - Bowel and bladder functions
  - Sleep
  - Lactation
  - Any ailment.

General

- Examination of/for
  - Fever
  - Anemia
  - Breast
  - Uterus
  - Lochia
  - TPR, BP, Pallor on examination.

- **Specific Examination**
  Note the size of the uterus
  Record the involution of the uterus

Sl No.	*Wk / Days*	*Involution – UT*	*Achieved Sig Yes No*
1.	Immediately following the delivery	At 20 wks of pregnancy	
2.	First 24 hrs	In the same position	
3.	First 2-3 days	Comes below umbilicus at the rate of 1 inch/day	
4.	3-6 days	Comes below at the rate of ½ inch/day	
5.	7-10 days	Descends beneath symphysis pubis and enters the pelvic cavity	
6.	Within 6 wks	UT regains its original size	

Inference: Normal Involution/Abnormal

- Note the smell and colours of lochia
- Examine episiotomy for healing process
- Look for s/s fever, breast complaints, pain in abdomen, fullness of abdomen, foul smelling discharge subinvolution and manage appropriately.

Aims of Second Postnatal Visit

- Study the involution of uterus
- Assess Hb levels
- Screen for fitness for contraception.

15

Management of Normal Peurperium

- Encourage the mother to ambulate (avoid strenuous activities)
- Educate the mother on the following:
  - Maintenance of personal perinatal hygiene
  - Advice light diet on the first day and subsequently can take normal diet
  - The mother should consume 300 kcal more than the non-lactating woman
  - Advise roughage rich diet
  - Encourage mother to pass urine frequently (4-6 hourly)
  - Episiotomy wound/stitches should be cleaned daily and dressed with antiseptic powder and covered with sterile pad
  - Encourage mother to change her diapers every 4-6 hrs
  - Educate the mother to wash her hand each time before feeding her baby
- Administer IFA tablets 6 mo. postpartum
- Advice abstinence for 6 wks
- Consume 550 kcl extra during lactating period
- Educate on child care.

Postpartum Minor Ailments and Mangement

Sl No.	*Minor ailment*	*Management*
1.	After pain (for 2-4 days)	Re-assurance Mild analgesics
2.	Retention of urine	Hot/cold water application on suprapubic region
3.	Pain (episiotomy site)	Tab/Ibuprofen 400 mg 8 hrly × 3-4 days
4.	Engorgement of breast	Hot water fomentation Light massage from periphery to nipple 5 units of syntocinon IM, may be given-following manual expression of milk
5.	Constipation	Roughage rich diet

Postpartum Problems/ Complications/Management

Problem	*S/S*	*Investigations*	*Management*
PUERPERAL PYREXIA TEMP 100° - 104°F within 14 days	Causes : • Puerperal sepsis • UTI • Breast engorgement and infection	• Hb • TLC • DLC • Urine for pus cells	**Prophylactic:** **AN period:** • Improve health and nutrition • Abstinence in the last 6 wks • Personal hygiene

Contd...

Contd...

Problem	*S/S*	*Investigations*	*Management*
of delivery	• Deep vein thrombosis		• Avoid infection **Intrapartum period** • Observe principles of cleanliness • Avoid unnecessary PV examinations • Treat injury of birth canal appropriately • Prescribe prophylactic antibiotics **Postpartum period** • Advise personal hygiene • Avoidance of too many visitors **Treatment** • Bed rest with head end raised to facilitate uterine discharge • Advice plenty of oral fluids • Prescribe appropriate antibiotics, e.g. Ampicillin 500 mg 6 hrly and metronidazole 400 mg 8 hrly

Contd...

Contd...

Problem	*S/S*	*Investigations*	*Management*
			• Administer methergine to promote uterine contraction
PUERPERAL SEPSIS Infection of the genital tract between onset of rupture of membranes labour and within 6 wks following delivery	• Fever with malaise • Temp 38-50°C • Abnormal vaginal discharge • Pelvic pain • Subinvolution of uterus • Vomiting • Headache • Tachycardia • Flushed face • PV shows tender parametrium and uterus	• >TLC • High Polymorphs levels • Hb levels • Vaginal discharge for C/S	• Bed rest • Plenty of oral fluids • Hydrotherapy • Antibiotics • Ref to FRU for further management

Contd...

15

Contd...

Problem	*S/S*	*Investigations*	*Management*
UTI	• Fever • Pain in Renal angle • H/O frequency of micturation • Dysuria • Retention of urine	• WBC count • Polymorph count • Urine has pus cells • Urine for c/s (+ve)	• Plenty of fluids • Antibiotics according to the sensitivity
BREAST ENGORGEMENT "due to exaggerated venous and Lymphatic enlargement Usually on 3rd or 4th postpartum-day	• Tense and tender breast • Knobby to feel • Fever • Pain		• Firm breast support • Cold fomentation • Pain killers • Expression of milk- Manually or by using breast pump

Contd...

Contd...

Problem	*S/S*	*Investigations*	*Management*
CRACKED NIPPLE Raw or loss of surface epithelium at the top or base of the nipple	CAUSE Due to unclean hygiene resulting in formation of crust over the nipple by retracted nipple/ vigorous sucking in engorged breast (or) Improper ways of breast feeding		Application of allantoin ointment if available or edible oil
ACUTE MASTITIS due to infection in a cracked nipple	CAUSE : • Infection by *Staphylococcus aureus* • Seen in 1st or 2nd wk of peurperium		• Treat using appropriate antibiotics • Administer sedatives • Avoid breast feeding on the affected side • Manual expression of milk from

Contd...

Contd...

Problem	*S/S*	*Investigations*	*Management*
	• Fever 102°F or more • Chills • Pain and swelling in one quadrant of the breast • Over-lying skin is hot and red • If left may lead to breast abscess		opposite side during feeding will be helpful
BREAST ABSCESS exhibited by fever at the end of the 1st wk	• Pain in breast • Cracked nipple • Temp 102°F 103°F • Localized tenderness	• WBC and Polymorph are high	• Breast support • Avoidance of breast feeding on the affected side • Appropriate antibiotics

Contd...

Contd...

Problem	*S/S*	*Investigations*	*Management*
	• Localized redness • Swelling in the breast		• Drainage of pus under general anaesthesia • If required ref to FRU
PUERPERAL VENOUS THROMBOSIS includes 1. Superficial thrombophlebitis 2. Deep-vein thrombosis	Predisposing factors 1. Anemia 2. Heart disease 3. Immobilization 4. Trauma 5. Local infection 6. Caesarian section 7. Use of oestrogens to suppress lactation	Affected area is painful, tender and red • The area is warm to touch with rapid pulse • Calf muscle pain positive homan sign • Positive humans signs	• Ref to FRU
PUERPERAL PSYCHOSIS	Predisposing factors	• Refusal of foods • Confusion	• Ref to FRU • Counsel

Contd..

Contd...

Problem	*S/S*	*Investigations*	*Management*
	1. Severe eclampsia 2. Difficult labour 3. Puerperal fever. The condition starts after 3-4 days of child birth as • insomnia • delusion	• Tendency to suicide • Tendency to infanticide	the relatives
POST-PARTUM HAEMORRHAGE	• H/O severe blood loss after delivery • H/O retained placenta • H/O instrumentation manipulation		PRIMARY MANAGEMENT • Treatment of shock • Oxytocics • Compression of tools • Suture of cervical and vaginal tears • Vaginal packing • Ref in left lateral position *Refer for:*

Contd...

Contd...

Problem	*S/S*	*Investigations*	*Management*
	during delivery • Hypovolaemic shock • Atonic UT • Tears in vagina, cervix on P/V examination		• Blood transfusions • Manual removal of placenta • Repair of tears in vaginal cervix
PUERPERAL SEPSIS	• History of fever with any of the following H/O foul smelling vaginal discharge • Abdominal tenderness • Pelvic or abdominal pain • Subinvolution of uterus		PRIMARY MANAGEMENT • Antibiotics • Refer to surgical intervention drainage REFER FOR • Investigations for c/s • Removal of retained products • Treatment of septic shock • Laparotomy is required

Contd...

DANGER SIGNS – PERINATAL PERIOD

Antenatal	*Intranatal*	*Postnatal*
• Fits • Passing fluid/ discharge from vagina (Amniotic fluid) • Headache • Visual disturbances • Bleeding PV with or (APH) without pain • Swelling of feet face, hands • Severe anemia • Any other unusual complaints	• Fits • Foetal distress • Malpresentations • No progress of labour for 12 hrs • Sluggish pains/No pains after rupture of membranes • Good pains following ROM, but poor progress of labour • Prolapse of the cord/hand • Meconium stained liquor • Slow, irregular, fast foetal heart rate • Excessive show or bleeding • Collapse during labour • Placenta not separated within ½ an hour	• Fits • Excessive Bleeding • Fever, Chills • Foul smelling vaginal discharge • Puerperal sepsis • Thrombophlebitis • UTI • Mastitis • PPH • Maternal exhaustion • Fever >38°C • S/S toxemia • Rising pulse rate

CHAPTER 16

Abortion

DEFINITION

Expulsion of products of conception before 20 wks is termed as abortion.

TYPES, DIAGNOSIS, MANAGEMENT

Furnished in tabular column.

No.	Symptoms	Threatened	Inevitable	Incomplete	Septic	Missed	Complete
A	History of amenorrhoea	Present	Present	Present	Present	Present	Present
B.	Vaginal bleeding	Scanty bright red or blood stained discharge	Frank bleeding; it may be severe at times	Continuous or recurrent bleeding	Foul smelling discharge	Nil or dirty brown or sanguin-ous discharge	May be present
C.	Abdominal pain	Commonly absent or slight, vague pain on back back and lower abdomen	Severe colicky pains in the lower abdomen	Abdominal pain may or may not be present	Pain may or may not be present. Later on with spread of infec-tion to the pelvic	Pain is absent	Present

Contd...

Contd...

No.	Symptoms	Threatened	Inevitable	Incomplete	Septic	Missed	Complete
					peri-toneum, severe pain in the lower abdomen		
D.	History of expulsion of the product of conception per vagina	Nil	Nil	Present	May or may not be present	Nil	Present
E.	Constitu-tional symptoms	Nil	May be present tachy-cardia, Low BP in case of	In severe blood loss, tachycardia, pallor, low BP, symp-toms of	Fever with chill is present, nausea vomiting	Absent	Absent

Contd...

Contd...

No.	Symptoms	Threatened	Inevitable	Incomplete	Septic	Missed	Complete
			heavy blood loss	shock may be present	may be present oliguria		
F.	Size uterus	Corresponding period of gestation	May be corresponding	Smaller than period of gestation	May be small with tenderness	Smaller than gestation	Smaller than period of gestation and Os closed
	Status of internal Os	Closed	Open	Open in recent and closed in old	May be closed	Os closed	
G.	Character of vaginal discharge	Scanty bleeding	Frank blood and clots	Recent or old blood (dark brown)	Foul smelling purulent puslike discharge	Thin brown or serosanguinous	Scanty fresh bleeding or no bleeding

Contd...

Contd...

No.	Symptoms	Threatened	Inevitable	Incomplete	Septic	Missed	Complete
					may be present	discharge may be present	
H.	Complications	May become inevitable or missed abortion	May become complete abortion, develop haemorrhagic shock, may become septic if handled by untrained persons	May become septic abortion, can develop anaemia	Maternal death, renal failure, endotoxis shock, septicemia, DIC (disseminated intra vascular coagulopathy)	Coagulation failure	No complication if no interference

Contd...

Contd...

No.	*Symptoms*	*Threatened*	*Inevitable*	*Incomplete*	*Septic*	*Missed*	*Complete*
I.	Investigations	Hb, urine for albumin and sugar	Hb, urine for albumin and sugar	Hb, urine for albumin and sugar	Hb, urine for albumin and sugar, DLC,TLC	Hb, urine for albumin and sugar, BT,CT, CRT	Hb%, urine alb. and sugar
J.	Treatment	Bed rest, abstinence, folic acid (1 mg) daily. Reevaluation after 4 wks or earlier in case of increased bleeding per	Resuscitation with IV fluids, evacuation of the uterus by suction, evacuation, injection Ergome-	Suction curettage is to be done if the external os is open. Dilatation of cervix followed by blunt	Hospitalize the patient. Start - Metronidazole, ampicillin, Gentamicin,	If the uterus is <10 wks size then suction evacuation may be done. If more than 10	No treatment is required if you have inspected the products. If not sure of

Contd...

Contd...

No.	Symptoms	Threatened	Inevitable	Incomplete	Septic	Missed	Complete
		vaginum or pain in lower abdomen	trine 0.2 mg IV followed by curettage If uterus is more than 12 wks and bleeding is severe, start syntocinon drip and refer to FRU	curettage is to be done if external os is closed If the uterus is more than 12 wks then refer to FRU as in inevitable abortion	parenterally. If the os is open uterus is < 10 wks then evacuate after 24 hrs of antibiotics or earlier if she bleeds. No curettage only digital	wks patient to be referred to FRU	the completeness do curettage dilatation may not be required

Contd...

Contd...

No.	*Symptoms*	*Threatened*	*Inevitable*	*Incomplete*	*Septic*	*Missed*	*Complete*
					evacuation is to be done. Monitor for complication and refer accordingly		

(Reproduced from the Module for Medical Officer, Inst. of National Health and Family Welfare)

CHAPTER 17

Contraception/ Fertility Regulation

DEFINITION

Contraceptive methods are defined as a set of methods adopted by women to avoid unwanted pregnancies.

Characteristics of a Good Contraceptive Method

A good contraceptive method is/are:
- Safe
- Effective
- Acceptable
- In expensive
- Reversible
- Simple to administer
- Requires little or no medical supervision.

Types of Contraceptive Methods

1. Temporary Contraceptive Methods (Spacing Methods).
2. Permanent Contraceptive Methods (Terminal Methods).

Contraception/Fertility Regulation

1. Spacing Methods

- A. Barrier
  - → Physical methods
    - → Condom
    - → Diaphragm
    - → Vaginal sponge
  - → Chemical methods
    - → Foams
    - → Creams, Jellies
    - → Suppositories
    - → Soluble films
  - → Combined methods
- B. Intrauterine devices
  - → I Generation devices → Lippes loop
  - → II Generation devices → Cu 'T' & ML devices
  - → III Generation devices → IUD with hormones
- C. Hormonal contraceptive → Oral pills
  - → Combined pills
  - → POP
  - → Postcoital pills (contraception)
  - → Once a month pill
  - → Male pill
- D. Post-conceptional methods
  - → Menstrual regulation
  - → Menstrual induction
- E. Miscellaneous
  - → Abstinence
  - → Coitus interrupts
  - → Calendar method
  - → Natural family planning methods
  - → Breast feeding
  - → Birth control vaccine

2. Terminal methods

- → Male sterilization
- → Female sterilization

CHAPTER 18

Sample Nursing Care Plans

NURSING CARE PLANS FOR A CHILD WITH FEVER

Name :

Classification of beneficiary : infant/ toddler/pre-schooler/schooler

Age :

Sex : M/F Level of prevention :- primary/ secondary/tertiary

Subjective/ objective data	*Nursing diagnosis*	*Objective*	*Interventions*	*Rationale*	*Evaluation/ outcomes*
SD : mother complaints that the child is unusually warm today	Alteration in body temperature (pyrexia) related to infection	Short term goal Attain normal body temp	1. Assess TPR/ Every 2 hrs as required	Assessment helps to manage the case appropriately	Temp is reduced (e.g.) 99°F after antipyretic and

Contd...

Contd...

Subjective/ objective data	*Nursing diagnosis*	*Objective*	*Interventions*	*Rationale*	*Evaluation/ outcomes*
					general intervention
OD : On observation child appears restless, on touch body is warm.		Long term goal Prevent further episodes of fever	2. Administer anti-pyretics, and antibiotics if required	Reduces the body temp	
			3. Assess the bowel pattern	Sometimes GI infections may accompany with signs of fever	Mother continues breast feeding

Contd...

Contd...

Subjective/ objective data	*Nursing diagnosis*	*Objective*	*Interventions*	*Rationale*	*Evaluation/ outcomes*
			4. Encourage mother to administer plenty of fluids, at frequent intervals	Helps in maintaining hydration, as water is lost in elevated temperature	—
			5. Advice the mother to continue breast feeding	Helps in combating infection to some extent. Breast milk is easily digestable	—

Contd...

Contd...

Subjective/ objective data	*Nursing diagnosis*	*Objective*	*Interventions*	*Rationale*	*Evaluation/ outcomes*
			6. Advice soft solid, non-greasy and non-oily diet	Bulky feeds, take long time for digestion	—
			7. Encourage the mother to dress the child with loose cotton garments	Helps is warding away the temperature	—
			8. Advice the mother to keep the	Helps in infection control and	—

Contd...

Contd...

Subjective/ objective data	*Nursing diagnosis*	*Objective*	*Interventions*	*Rationale*	*Evaluation/ outcomes*
			room, house adequately ventilated	facilitates convection of the temperature	
			9. Advocate tepid sponge, ice pack, if required	If temp is below 100°F, primary measures, like these help in maintaining	
			10. Health educate the mother on CSP (Cause,	Helps in preventing further episodes of	Mother verbalises the causes of fever

Contd...

Contd...

Subjective/ objective data	*Nursing diagnosis*	*Objective*	*Interventions*	*Rationale*	*Evaluation/ outcomes*
			Spread and Prevention) of fever	fever	
			11. Take relevant management steps if the temperature raise is due to ARI or depending on the specific cause	Raise of temp is often a prodromal sign for ARI/ Diarrhoea	

Contd...

Contd...

Subjective/ objective data	*Nursing diagnosis*	*Objective*	*Interventions*	*Rationale*	*Evaluation/ outcomes*
			12. Advice the mother not to take the child to crowded places or allow people with infection to handle the child	Helps in prevention of infection	Mother promises to abide by advice

Contd...

Contd...

Subjective/ objective data	*Nursing diagnosis*	*Objective*	*Interventions*	*Rationale*	*Evaluation/ outcomes*
			13. Educate the mother to dress the child according to seasonal variation	—	

NURSING CARE PLANS FOR A CHILD WITH DIARRHOEA

Name :

Classification of beneficiary : infant/toddler/preschooler/schooler

Age :

Sex : M/F Level of prevention: primary/secondary/tertiary

Subjective/ objective data	*Nursing diagnosis*	*Objective*	*Interventions*	*Rationale*	*Evaluation/ outcomes*
SD: Mother complains of frequent loose stools since morning	Alteration in bowel pattern (Diarrhoea) related to GI infection	Short term goal: restore hydration status	1. Assess the level of dehydration and assess TPR	Hydration status helps in deciding the management	

Contd...

Contd...

Subjective/ objective data	*Nursing diagnosis*	*Objective*	*Interventions*	*Rationale*	*Evaluation/ outcomes*
OD: on observations child looks dull and dehydrated		Long term goal: prevent further episodes of diarrhoea	2. Assess the stool (colour, consistency, frequency, odour)	Gives clue on kind/ cause of diarrhoea and helps in appropriate management	
			3. Enquire on the food intake previous 24 hrs	Aids in arriving at appropriate diagnosis	

Contd...

Contd...

Subjective/ objective data	*Nursing diagnosis*	*Objective*	*Interventions*	*Rationale*	*Evaluation/ outcomes*
			4. Administer ORS if mild dehydration is present	Corrects dehydration	The child is hydrated adequacy
			5. Advocate home available fluids are recommended (rice water with salt)	HAF are safe, effective and easily available	

Contd...

Contd...

Subjective/ objective data	*Nursing diagnosis*	*Objective*	*Interventions*	*Rationale*	*Evaluation/ outcomes*
			6. If dehydration is severe refer to FRU	Severe cases needs to be managed in care settings	
			7. Depending on the hydration status, presence/ absence of vomiting with diarrhoea advice feeds	Vomiting rapidly results in dehydration	

Contd...

Contd...

Subjective/ objective data	*Nursing diagnosis*	*Objective*	*Interventions*	*Rationale*	*Evaluation/ outcomes*
			8. Continue breast feeding if the child is on breast feed	Breast milk is contamination free, safe and aids in hydration	
			9. Advocate more of fluid diets	Maintains hydration	
			10. Advice soft solid carbohydrate based diet	Easily digestible	

Contd...

Contd...

Subjective/ objective data	*Nursing diagnosis*	*Objective*	*Interventions*	*Rationale*	*Evaluation/ outcomes*
			11. Avoid wheat and protein diets, roughage diet	Encourages rapid multiplication of bacterial load in the gut and complicated digestive process	
			12. Administer antibiotics relevant to the assess-	Antibiotic checks infection by acting upon the micro-	

Contd...

Contd...

Subjective/ objective data	*Nursing diagnosis*	*Objective*	*Interventions*	*Rationale*	*Evaluation/ outcomes*
			ment and the status of the child	organisms	
			13. General advice on the following a. General cleanliness b. Feeding cleanliness c. Disposal of stools	Helps in apt management and in preventing further episodes of diarrhoea	Mother verbalizes the importance of cleanliness, cause, spread and prevention of diarrhoea

Contd...

Contd...

Subjective/ objective data	*Nursing diagnosis*	*Objective*	*Interventions*	*Rationale*	*Evaluation/ outcomes*
			d. Hygiene of napkins e. Care while introducing weaning foods f. Discourage bottle feeds		
			14. Health education/(H/E on the afore stated points including	Helps in apt management and in preventing further epi-	

Contd...

Contd...

Subjective/ objective data	*Nursing diagnosis*	*Objective*	*Interventions*	*Rationale*	*Evaluation/ outcomes*
			cause, spread and prevention of diarrhoea	sodes of diarrhoea	
			15. Demonstrate specific diet preparations e.g. a. Rice-fried channa conjee b. Arraroot conjee	Helps in appropriate dietary management of diarrhoea	Mother demonstrates the preparation of conjee

Contd...

Contd...

Subjective/ objective data	*Nursing diagnosis*	*Objective*	*Interventions*	*Rationale*	*Evaluation/ outcomes*
			16. Administer vit 'A' regularly at an interval of 6 months	Improves defence activity be strengthening the lining epithelium of gut	

NURSING CARE PLAN FOR A CHILD WITH ACUTE RESPIRATORY INFECTION

Name :

Classification of beneficiary: infant/toddler/pre-schooler/schooler

Age:

Sex : M/F Level of Prevention : primary/secondary/tertiary

Subjective/ objective data	*Nursing diagnosis*	*Objective*	*Interventions*	*Rationale*	*Evaluation/ outcomes*
SD: Mother complaints that the child has running nose	Alteration in breathing pattern related to respiratory infection (Tachypnoea)	Short term goal: Achieve normal breathing pattern	1. Assess ARI	Assessment helps in managing accordingly	

Contd...

Contd...

Subjective/ objective data	*Nursing diagnosis*	*Objective*	*Interventions*	*Rationale*	*Evaluation/ outcomes*
OD: Child appears restless and dyspneic		Long term goal Prevent further episodes of ARI	2. Auscultate the chest for abnormal breathing sounds	Suggests information on respiratory system pathology and secretions	
			3. Advocate steam inhalation for the child along with the mother	Loosens the thick secretions	The child is able to breath, freely following the steam inhalation

Contd...

Contd...

Subjective/ objective data	*Nursing diagnosis*	*Objective*	*Interventions*	*Rationale*	*Evaluation/ outcomes*
			4. Do chest cuffing to loosen the secretions (phlem) following steam inhalation	Loosens the thick secretions	
			5. Encourage fluid intake	Helps in hydration and liquefaction of secretions	

Contd...

Contd...

Subjective/ objective data	*Nursing diagnosis*	*Objective*	*Interventions*	*Rationale*	*Evaluation/ outcomes*
			6. Advice protective clothings (sweaters, woolen clothings)	Offers protection against developing ARI	
			7. Advice the mother to serve warm fluids and foods/in small quan-	Prevents constriction of tracheobronchial tree which is already plugged with secretions	

Contd...

Contd...

Subjective/ objective data	*Nursing diagnosis*	*Objective*	*Interventions*	*Rationale*	*Evaluation/ outcomes*
			tities and continue breast feeding		
			8. Raise the head end of the child, while sleeping using pillows	Helps the child to freely breath, as this avoid abdominal viscera compressing against the diaphragm	

Contd...

Contd...

Subjective/ objective data	Nursing diagnosis	Objective	Interventions	Rationale	Evaluation/ outcomes
			9. Avoid tight clothings	Facilitates free breathing	
			10. Keep the house well ventilated at the same time warm by room heaters, etc.	Helps in preventing ARI by maintenance of general hygiene and warmth of the surrounding air	
			11. Advice the mother to	Such practices as these helps	

Contd...

Contd...

Subjective/ objective data	*Nursing diagnosis*	*Objective*	*Interventions*	*Rationale*	*Evaluation/ outcomes*
			administer, practicable home remedies such as honey with pepper, powder milk with turmeric	in loosening the secretions and improves ciliary action of the lining epithelium of the respiratory tract	
			12. Administer antibiotics and anti-	Helps in combating infection	

Contd...

Contd...

Subjective/ objective data	*Nursing diagnosis*	*Objective*	*Interventions*	*Rationale*	*Evaluation/ outcomes*
			pyretics if required as relevant to age and condition of the child		
			13. Advice the mother to maintain the general hygiene of the house and the immediate environment	Prevents episodes of ARI	

Contd...

Contd...

Subjective/ objective data	*Nursing diagnosis*	*Objective*	*Interventions*	*Rationale*	*Evaluation/ outcomes*
			14. H/E the mother on CSP of ARI	Improves the mothers knowledge and hence can help in preventing ARI episodes	Mother verbalizes the CSP of ARI
			15. Administer Vit 'A' periodically at an interval of 6 months	Strengthens the functioning of the lining epithelium of the respiratory tract	Mother promises to administer Vit 'A' periodically

NURSING CARE OF AN UNDER WEIGHT CHILD

Name :

Classification of beneficiary : infant/ toddler/pre-schooler/schooler

Age :

Sex : M/F Level of Prevention: primary/secondary/tertiary

Subjective/ objective data	*Nursing diagnosis*	*Objective*	*Interventions*	*Rationale*	*Evaluation/ outcomes*
SD: Mother complaints that her child gains weight poorly	Alteration in body mass (under weight) due to faulty feeding practices or worm infestation	Short term goal Treat for worm infestation / correct feeding practice	1. Assess the anthropometry of the child (Height, Weight, MAC,CC, HC & skin fold thickness)	Anthropometry serves as an important tool, to assess and plan the nutritional rehabilitation	

Contd...

Contd...

Subjective/ objective data	*Nursing diagnosis*	*Objective*	*Interventions*	*Rationale*	*Evaluation/ outcomes*
OD: On appearance the child looks thin and weak for the age		Long term goal Improve the weight of the child	2. Perform physical assessment of the child assess for pica eating	Physical assessment may reveal nutritional deficiency states, e.g. Bitot spot	
			3. If records are available assess the pattern of weight gain	Helps in understanding the child's weight gain pattern	

Contd...

Contd...

Subjective/ objective data	*Nursing diagnosis*	*Objective*	*Interventions*	*Rationale*	*Evaluation/ outcomes*
			4. Get more information of passing worms in the stools	Helps to confirm the cause of poor weight gain if it is due to worm infestation	
			5. Obtain general history of infection of the child, i.e. no. of episodes of	Serves as indicator and helps to assess the cause of poor weight gain	Child exhibits 4-5 episodes of infection in a year

Contd...

Contd...

Subjective/ objective data	*Nursing diagnosis*	*Objective*	*Interventions*	*Rationale*	*Evaluation/ outcomes*
			ARI (diarrhoea, etc.)		
			6. Get detailed information on the dietary pattern and food habits of the family and specifically the child's food habit	Helps in planning and chalking out sample menu and in advising menu plan	

Contd...

Contd...

Subjective/ objective data	*Nursing diagnosis*	*Objective*	*Interventions*	*Rationale*	*Evaluation/ outcomes*
			7. Deworm the child (Mebandazole- 400 mg X (Zentil, worm out) single dose once in 6 months		Child passed worms in the stool
			8. Introduce the concept of small frequent meals / snacks with	Helps in building up weight	

Contd...

Contd...

Subjective/ objective data	*Nursing diagnosis*	*Objective*	*Interventions*	*Rationale*	*Evaluation/ outcomes*
			plenty of fruits and vegetables		
			9. Educate and demonstrate the preparation of nutritious food items, such as the nutritious balls, Fe+ rich snack items like burfi, pulses dosa,	Helps in effective implementation when the mother is actively participating in the rehabilitation plan	Mother demonstrates the preparation of diet

Contd...

Contd...

Subjective/ objective data	*Nursing diagnosis*	*Objective*	*Interventions*	*Rationale*	*Evaluation/ outcomes*
			etc. (advice protein rich diet)		
			10. Advice vitamin supplements along with nutritional rehabilitation	Helps additionally to increase the weight	
			11. Advice and educate the mother on the	Mother's participation ensures her commitment	Mother promises to monitor the weight of the child

Contd...

Contd...

Subjective/ objective data	*Nursing diagnosis*	*Objective*	*Interventions*	*Rationale*	*Evaluation/ outcomes*
			concept of weight monitoring and means to improve the weight of the child (Maintenance of growth chart)	in the child care	
			12. Suggest plan sample menu / rehabilitation	Helps the family to scientifically participate	

Contd...

Contd...

Subjective/ objective data	*Nursing diagnosis*	*Objective*	*Interventions*	*Rationale*	*Evaluation/ outcomes*
			menu for the child keeping in mind the socioeconomic condition of the child	in the weight gain process	

NURSING CARE PLAN FOR A CHILD WITH DELAYED MILESTONE

Name :

Classification of beneficiary : infant / toddler / pre-schooler / schooler

Age :

Sex : M/F Level of Prevention : primary / secondary / tertiary

Subjective/ objective data	*Nursing diagnosis*	*Objective*	*Interventions*	*Rationale*	*Evaluation/ outcomes*
SD: Mother complains that the child has not got its dentition (the child is	Alteration in growth pattern (delayed milestone) related to faulty feeding practices	**Long term goal** attain the normal developmental milestone	1. Carry out physical assessment 2. Perform anthro-	Assessment reveals the status of milestone Faltering anthropometry may suggest	

Contd...

Contd...

Subjective/ objective data	*Nursing diagnosis*	*Objective*	*Interventions*	*Rationale*	*Evaluation/ outcomes*
1 yr 2 months)			pometry of the child	abnormalities in developmental milestone	
OD: On observation child looks weak and dentition not achieved			3. Assess the dietary pattern and food habits of the child	Helps in assessing the cause and suggesting remedial diet plan	

Contd...

Contd...

Subjective/ objective data	*Nursing diagnosis*	*Objective*	*Interventions*	*Rationale*	*Evaluation/ outcomes*
			4. Assess the developmental milestone of the child		
			5. Educate the mother on nutritional intervention (as specified for care of a child with under weight) focus	Most of the delayed milestones are often associated with faulty dietary pattern	

Contd...

Contd...

Subjective/ objective data	*Nursing diagnosis*	*Objective*	*Interventions*	*Rationale*	*Evaluation/ outcomes*
			on specific nutrients / as needed		
			6. Educate the mother on the normal developmental milestones and the importance of monitoring	Empowers the mother with sufficient and necessary education to participate in child care	

Contd...

Contd...

Subjective/ objective data	*Nursing diagnosis*	*Objective*	*Interventions*	*Rationale*	*Evaluation/ outcomes*
			7. Provide the mother with ready reckoner for developmental milestone so that she can monitor the milestone of her child	Helps the mother to monitor her child's developmental milestone	

SIMILAR OTHER NURSING CARE PLANS CAN BE DRAFTED UNDER FOLLOWING HEADINGS / CONDITIONS FOR U5

1. Breast Feeding
2. Growth Monitoring
3. Immunization
4. Weaning / supplementary diet
5. Developmental milestone
6. Prevention of accidents
7. Deworming / Vit 'A' Supplementation / Fe+ Supplementation
8. Reading / Writing / Learning Educational Skills
9. Care during illness, Cord care, Play therapies, etc.
10. Care of differently abled and HIV children.

NURSING CARE PLAN – ANTENATAL MOTHER

Name :

Classification of beneficiary : infant / toddler/ pre-schooler / schooler /AN/ PN/Adult/others

Age :

Sex : M/F Level of Prevention :- primary / secondary / tertiary

Subjective/ objective data	*Nursing diagnosis*	*Objective*	*Interventions*	*Rationale*	*Evaluation/ outcomes*
SD : Mrs x.... married since 1 yr gives history of aminorrhea for a month	Pregnancy	Provide routine and specific Antenatal care (Refer antenatal care)	1. Subject the mother to GRAVINDEX test	Confirms pregnancy	

Contd:...

Contd...

Subjective/ objective data	*Nursing diagnosis*	*Objective*	*Interventions*	*Rationale*	*Evaluation/ outcomes*
OD : will be subjected to routine investigations			2. Register the mother with the local health unit HSC, PHC, tertiary hospital as relevant	Helps in promptly monitoring the pregnancy	Write relevant outcomes and improvements depending on interventions
			3. Collect general and specific antenatal history	Helps in designing AN care	

Contd...

Contd...

Subjective/ objective data	*Nursing diagnosis*	*Objective*	*Interventions*	*Rationale*	*Evaluation/ outcomes*
			4. Carry out the following investigations: Ht, Wt, Vital signs, Blood grouping, Typing, U/S, U/A, Breast examination VDRL	Helps in designing AN care accordingly	
		Immunization	5. Administer 1st Dose of TT on confirmation of	Confers immunity against	

Contd...

Contd...

Subjective/ objective data	*Nursing diagnosis*	*Objective*	*Interventions*	*Rationale*	*Evaluation/ outcomes*
			pregnancy 2nd Dose 1 month apart from 1 dose for Primi	tetanus (for Pregnancy) within 3 yrs, 1 dose TT is sufficient Helps in management of minor ailments in pregnancy	
			6. Advocate healthy diet and provide tips in	Due to HCG in the blood. Generally settles down	

Contd...

Contd...

Subjective/ objective data	*Nursing diagnosis*	*Objective*	*Interventions*	*Rationale*	*Evaluation/ outcomes*
			management of minor ailments		
			• Nausea / vomiting – usually self limiting and receeds and settles down by 3 months	Is due to compression of the bladder due to distension/ enlargement of UT	
			• Frequency of micturation	Due to compression	

Contd...

18

Contd...

Subjective/ objective data	*Nursing diagnosis*	*Objective*	*Interventions*	*Rationale*	*Evaluation/ outcomes*
			– self limiting by 3 months	of the rectum, due to enlargement of UT	
			• Constipation – encourage more of fluid diet, increase roughage in the diet	Is experienced due to indigestion. Avoid full meals	
			• Heart burn – advocate bland diet.	The enlarging abdomen	

Contd...

Contd...

Subjective/ objective data	*Nursing diagnosis*	*Objective*	*Interventions*	*Rationale*	*Evaluation/ outcomes*
			Avoid spicy diets, if excessive administer antacid • Dyspnoea – to wear loose garments facilitating easy breathing. Generally experienced	compress the diaphragm and hence reduces the superior – inferior diameter of the thorax, resulting in dyspnoea	

Contd...

Contd...

Subjective/ objective data	*Nursing diagnosis*	*Objective*	*Interventions*	*Rationale*	*Evaluation/ outcomes*
		Management of warning signs	• The following warning signs are to be detected and managed approximately		
			• Blurring of vision, excessive oedema, sudden / excessive weight – gain (>10-12 kg throughout	(Ref. AN care) The warning signs are vital indicators of the forthcoming	

Contd...

Contd...

Subjective/ objective data	*Nursing diagnosis*	*Objective*	*Interventions*	*Rationale*	*Evaluation/ outcomes*
			pregnancy), excessive tiredness, leaking / bleeding PV, pain abdomen, reduction / absence of fetal movements, these conditions to be explained to the mother and managed	complications and hence to be managed with due care	

Contd...

Contd...

Subjective/ objective data	*Nursing diagnosis*	*Objective*	*Interventions*	*Rationale*	*Evaluation/ outcomes*
			appropriately in FRU		
		Exercise, rest and sleep	• Advice regular house hold activities • Advocate 8 hrs sleep during day time compulsorily • Advice frequent rest while carry-	Sufficient exercise, rest and sleep is a must for healthy pregnancy	

Contd...

Contd...

Subjective/ objective data	*Nursing diagnosis*	*Objective*	*Interventions*	*Rationale*	*Evaluation/ outcomes*
			ing out house hold works • Mild, Antenatal exercises to be advocated. (Demonstrate AN exercises)		
		Diet / nutrition	• Assess the food pattern, dietary habits	Assessment helps in designing appropriate care	
			• Carry out 24		

Contd...

Contd...

Subjective/ objective data	*Nursing diagnosis*	*Objective*	*Interventions*	*Rationale*	*Evaluation/ outcomes*
			hrs recall • Compare the intake in terms of CHO, Protein, Fat, Fe+, Ca and KCal as against the recommended dietary allowances	Helps in scientifically devising / advising diet for the mother	
			• Design a sample	Helps in better	

Contd...

Contd...

Subjective/ objective data	*Nursing diagnosis*	*Objective*	*Interventions*	*Rationale*	*Evaluation/ outcomes*
			menu and educate the mother accordingly	nutrition of the mother	
			• Advocate and demonstrate items that are nutritious	Helps and promotes the nutritional status of the mother	
			• Keep in mind socioeconomic conditions of the mother while		

Contd...

Contd...

Subjective/ objective data	*Nursing diagnosis*	*Objective*	*Interventions*	*Rationale*	*Evaluation/ outcomes*
			advising on the diet		
			• Supplement regular calcium and iron / folic acid, from 3 month onwards • Advocate 2 glasses of milk every day	Promotes general health and especially caters tools the micro-nutrient needs of the women helps in easy digestion and	

Contd...

Contd...

Subjective/ objective data	*Nursing diagnosis*	*Objective*	*Interventions*	*Rationale*	*Evaluation/ outcomes*
			• Advice small frequent meals • Advocate easily digestable diet, avoid spicy oily and heavy diet	prevents heart burn and prevents fullness feeling	
		Check up	• Advice regular check ups as follows till 6 months, One visit a month	Helps in monitoring and ensuring an uneventful pregnancy	

Contd...

Contd...

Subjective/ objective data	*Nursing diagnosis*	*Objective*	*Interventions*	*Rationale*	*Evaluation/ outcomes*
			6-8 months – twice a month 8+ -every week		
		Preparation for delivery	• Advise the importance of regular visits, importance of getting AN card and relevant documents		

Contd...

Contd...

Subjective/ objective data	*Nursing diagnosis*	*Objective*	*Interventions*	*Rationale*	*Evaluation/ outcomes*
			• Advice on the importance of institutional delivery	Helps in preventing MMR	
			• Advice on the selection of place (hospital / Institution) for delivery especially for primi	In Indian context mothers generally opt to remain in their, mother's	

Contd...

Contd...

Subjective/ objective data	*Nursing diagnosis*	*Objective*	*Interventions*	*Rationale*	*Evaluation/ outcomes*
				house, i.e. a place other than regular visits	
			• Advice on the material preparation, financial preparation for the delivery	Helps in preventing unnecessary and unplanned expenditure	
		Monitoring vital parameters	Monitor the following in prescribed formats	Helps in monitoring pregnancy and	

Contd...

Contd...

Subjective/ objective data	*Nursing diagnosis*	*Objective*	*Interventions*	*Rationale*	*Evaluation/ outcomes*
			1. Weight Gain 2. Urine Sugar 3. Urine Albumin 4. Ca, Fe Supplementation 5. Immunization Status of the Mother 6. Other relevant uninformation, as pertinent. (Monitoring	detecting complications at the earliest and managing them appropriately	

Contd...

Contd...

Subjective/ objective data	*Nursing diagnosis*	*Objective*	*Interventions*	*Rationale*	*Evaluation/ outcomes*
			Fundal Height) Health educate the mother on the following • General hygiene • Prevention of infection • Management of anaemia • Immunization • Exercise, rest, sleep		

Contd...

Contd...

Subjective/ objective data	*Nursing diagnosis*	*Objective*	*Interventions*	*Rationale*	*Evaluation/ outcomes*
			• Nutrition and supplementation • Weaning signs • Contraception – family planning • Preparation for delivery • Newborn care • Care of infant – Colostrum feeding		

Contd...

Contd...

Subjective/ objective data	*Nursing diagnosis*	*Objective*	*Interventions*	*Rationale*	*Evaluation/ outcomes*
			- Avoidance of prelacteal feeds - Breast feeding - Weaning and supplementary diets - Growth monitoring - Immunization		
			• Postnatal care – Prevention of infection - General hygiene and	Helps in postnatal well being	

Contd...

Contd...

Subjective/ objective data	*Nursing diagnosis*	*Objective*	*Interventions*	*Rationale*	*Evaluation/ outcomes*
			perineal hygiene – Lochia etc. - Care of breast - Postnatal diet - Postnatal supplementation (Ca, Fa and Vit 'A') - Postnatal exercises - Any other as relevant (weaning		

Contd...

Contd...

Subjective/ objective data	*Nursing diagnosis*	*Objective*	*Interventions*	*Rationale*	*Evaluation/ outcomes*
			signs) like raise of temp, excessive bleeding, breast abscess, etc. **Note :** Also Ref AN care and incorporate relevant care components		

NURSING CARE PLAN – POSTNATAL MOTHER

Name : Classification of beneficiary : infant / toddler / pre-schooler / schooler / AN / PN / Morbidity condition (specify)

Age :

Level of Prevention : primary / secondary / tertiary

Subjective/ objective data	*Nursing diagnosis*	*Objective*	*Interventions*	*Rationale*	*Evaluation/ outcomes*
Postnatal mother	PN mother	PN care	• Obtain the following base line information - Type of delivery - Date of delivery - Delivery conducted by - Place of delivery (Home / Institution) - Apgar (for the child)	Helps in designing care	Implement care and record relevant outcomes

Contd...

Contd...

Subjective/ objective data	*Nursing diagnosis*	*Objective*	*Interventions*	*Rationale*	*Evaluation/ outcomes*
		Immediate postnatal care	- Vital signs (TPR) during delivery • Design and implement the following PN care • Educate the mother if she encounters any of the following and appropriately manage - Raise of temperature - Foul smelling lochia - Breast engorgement - Breast abscess - Problems in breast feeding (due to fiss-	Raise of temperature suggests infection, it may head to PN septicaemia and hence needs to be managed Bleeding PV	

Contd...

Contd...

Subjective/ objective data	*Nursing diagnosis*	*Objective*	*Interventions*	*Rationale*	*Evaluation/ outcomes*
			ured nipple, inverted / sore nipple, etc.) - Bleeding P/V	excessively, may be a case of PPH	
		Hygiene	• Advice general hygiene, including pereneal hygiene • Educate the mother on lochia and related physiological aspects • Advise pereneal wash with luke warm water twice a day • Educate and emphasize on care of episiotomy line	• Prevents infection • Helps the mother to appropriately manage	

Contd...

Contd...

Subjective/ objective data	*Nursing diagnosis*	*Objective*	*Interventions*	*Rationale*	*Evaluation/ outcomes*
			• Assess the nutritional pattern, dietary habits	• Helps in assessing and designing menu plan	
		Nutrition	• Perform 24 hrs recall • Compare actual intake with RDA • Devise a sample menu • Advice plenty of fluids, balanced diet, roughage diet	Increased fluid intake results in optimal urine out put and hence can purge organisms from pereneal region	
		Conventional	• Discourage the practice of conventional food items specifically practiced for the PN mothers		

Contd...

Contd...

Subjective/ objective data	*Nursing diagnosis*	*Objective*	*Interventions*	*Rationale*	*Evaluation/ outcomes*
			• Educate the importance of consuming all regular items	Roughage diet helps in avoiding constipation, which in any other wise result in straining and eventually result in gaping of the episiotomy would	
			• Advice supplementation of calcium, iron tablets and Vit 'A' solution	Supplementation helps both the mother and the child in meeting the macro and micronutrients.	
	Exercise, rest and sleep		• Advocate regular house hold activities • Encourage sufficient	Helps in maintaining general well being	

Contd...

Contd...

Subjective/ objective data	*Nursing diagnosis*	*Objective*	*Interventions*	*Rationale*	*Evaluation/ outcomes*
			rest and sleep • Teach postnatal exercises		
		Health education	• Advice and health educate the mother on the following: - Prevention of PN infections - General hygiene - Nutrition, supplementation - Rest , exercise and sleep - Involution of uterus	Aims at promoting material well being Aims at promoting infant well being, a healthy postnatal period	

Contd...

Contd...

Subjective/ objective data	*Nursing diagnosis*	*Objective*	*Interventions*	*Rationale*	*Evaluation/ outcomes*
			- Care of episiotomy wound - Contraception - Importance of breast feeding - Avoidance of prelacteal feeds - Weaning and supplementation - Growth monitoring - Immunization		
		Maintenance of relevant records	Maintain relevant records as follows, - Involution of uterus	Aims in monitoring and ensuring PN period	

Contd...

Contd...

Subjective/ objective data	*Nursing diagnosis*	*Objective*	*Interventions*	*Rationale*	*Evaluation/ outcomes*
			- Ca, Fe, and Vit 'A' Supplementation - BP, TPR - Postnatal check ups		

NURSING CARE PLAN – DIABETIC CLIENT

Name : Classification of beneficiary : infant / toddler / pre-schooler / schooler / AN / PN / Morbidity condition (specify)

Age :

Sex : M/F Level of Prevention : primary / secondary / tertiary

Subjective/objective data	*Nursing diagnosis*	*Objective*	*Interventions*	*Rationale*	*Evaluation/outcomes*
SD: Client complaints of dizziness and expresses having DM since 6 months		Diabetic Care	• Check blood glucose levels if required • Perform U/S and classify the client	Helps in confirming and designing the care	
	Alteration in blood glucose level (elevated blood glu-	Attain and maintain normal blood glucose level	Will be maintained by the following interventions.		

Contd...

Contd...

Subjective/ objective data	*Nursing diagnosis*	*Objective*	*Interventions*	*Rationale*	*Evaluation/outcomes*
OD:- Urine for sugar reveals presence of DM	cose) related to Diabetes Mellitus	by following sub objectives			
		Nutrition	• Assess the dietary pattern and food habits : assess locally available resources • Perform 24 hrs recall	Helps in deciding the sample menu	
			• Calculate the CHO, KCal and Fat contents and compare them with RDA	Helps in scientifically devising the food pattern	

Contd...

Contd...

Subjective/ objective data	*Nursing diagnosis*	*Objective*	*Interventions*	*Rationale*	*Evaluation/outcomes*
			• Draw inference and design a sample menu according to the pattern of life style (sedentary worker, light or heavy worker)	Helps the client to follow the diet scientifically	
			• Educate the client on foods to be included in plenty and foods to be avoided		
			• Prepare a list of the above said and give to the client	Helps in reinforcement of the knowledge given	
			• Advice and educate on the importance of	Irrespective of the pharmacological	

Contd...

Contd...

Subjective/ objective data	*Nursing diagnosis*	*Objective*	*Interventions*	*Rationale*	*Evaluation/outcomes*
			dietary modification and dietary management of blood glucose levels	management the dietary management helps pertinently in maintaining the blood glucose levels	
			• Assess the duration for which the client has been diabetic	Helps in deciding on managing the care and health education	
		Maintenance of glucose levels by pharmacological means	• Obtain history, on the existing pharmacological means of management, i.e. insulin or antidiabetic drugs		
			• If the client is an insulin dependant client, then	Helps in appropriate management	

Contd...

Contd...

Subjective/ objective data	*Nursing diagnosis*	*Objective*	*Interventions*	*Rationale*	*Evaluation/outcomes*
			obtain information as follows - Type of insulin Plain Lente - Units of insulin used - Self administered by health care professionals		
			• Teach the art-self administration and teach on the accessible sites	Helps the client to be independent and participate in self care	
			• Prepare a picture and chart it and hand it	Helps in reinforcement of the knowledge	

Contd...

Contd...

Subjective/ objective data	*Nursing diagnosis*	*Objective*	*Interventions*	*Rationale*	*Evaluation/outcomes*
			over to the client for easy reference	given	
			• Teach the aseptic techniques of injection administrations and dietary responsibilities following during insulin administration	Prevents injection abscess and avoids errors in medication and helps in adherence to therapeutic regime	
		In case of antidiabetics	• Maintain insulin chart as follows		
			• Obtain history of oral antidiabetics, e.g.	Helps in scientifically	

Insulin chart (within Interventions column):

Sl. no	Date	Time	Insulin	Units	Rem	Sig

Contd...

Contd...

Subjective/ objective data	*Nursing diagnosis*	*Objective*	*Interventions*	*Rationale*	*Evaluation/outcomes*
			Dianil/ glyciphage, etc. with dose and prescription	managing the client	
			• Educate the emphasis on the regular adherence to the therapeutic regimen	Effectively controls glucose levels, prevents complication by regular adherence	
			• Educate and explain on the accompanying responsibilities		
			• Monitor the strength of the drug and educate the client to	Promotes apt adherence to the prescriptions	

Contd...

Contd...

Subjective/ objective data	*Nursing diagnosis*	*Objective*	*Interventions*	*Rationale*	*Evaluation/outcomes*
			follow the prescribed dose • In both case check the prescription • Maintain drug chart as follows		
		Exercise	• Advocate, mild moderate exercises • Educate on the importance of regular exercise in maintaining general health status	Maintains and helps in regulation of BMR and in maintain blood	

Drug chart (within Interventions):

Sl. no	Date	Time	Drug	dose	Yes	No	Units	Rem	Sig

Contd...

Contd...

Subjective/ objective data	*Nursing diagnosis*	*Objective*	*Interventions*	*Rationale*	*Evaluation/outcomes*
				glucose levels	
		Prevention of complications	• Educate the client on probable complication (Cardiomyopathies, Nephropathy, Neuropathies, Diabetic Retinopathies, Diabetic Keto-acidosis, etc.)'	Helps the client to recognize the warning signs and seek medical help	
			• Educate on the presenting warning signs of complications like sweet odour, ketonuria, giddiness, etc.		
		(Ref Diabetic records)	• Emphasis on the need of possessing diabetic identity card for aid in	Helps in management during	
		Care of foot			

Contd...

Contd...

Subjective/ objective data	*Nursing diagnosis*	*Objective*	*Interventions*	*Rationale*	*Evaluation/outcomes*
			case of emergencies • Periodically assess the condition of feet • Advise usage of foot wear regular trimming and maintenance of nails	emergencies Helps in preventing cuts, injuries which takes along time to heal and predisposes the individual to develop gangrene	
		Health education	Health educate the client on the following • Importance of maintaining blood glucose levels	Helps in a complete participation of the client in his care and	

Contd...

Contd...

Subjective/ objective data	*Nursing diagnosis*	*Objective*	*Interventions*	*Rationale*	*Evaluation/outcomes*
			• Importance of adherence to therapeutic regimen and S/S over and under dosage • Dietary management of blood sugar levels • Regular exercises • Warning signs complication • S/S hypo- and hyperglycemia • Management during emergencies • Preventions and management of	therapy ensures: optional management	

Contd...

Contd...

Subjective/ objective data	*Nursing diagnosis*	*Objective*	*Interventions*	*Rationale*	*Evaluation/outcomes*
			complications • Foot care • Foods to be included and avoided • Importance of carrying diabetic ID card		

NURSING CARE PLAN FOR A HYPERTENSIVE CLIENT

Name : Classification of beneficiary : infant / toddler / pre-schooler / schooler / AN / PN / Morbidity condition(specify)

Age : Level of Prevention : primary / secondary / tertiary

Subjective/ objective data	*Nursing diagnosis*	*Objective*	*Interventions*	*Rationale*	*Evaluation/outcomes*
The client expresses that he is Hypertensive since 6 months	(Elevated blood pressure)	Maintain BP within acceptance range	Carryout the following intervention as per sub-objectives stated		
BP = $\geq \frac{140}{90}$		Promote adherence to thera-	• Obtain history of the client – duration of illness, details of	Serves as baseline data for	Implement and record

Contd...

Contd...

Subjective/ objective data	Nursing diagnosis	Objective	Interventions	Rationale	Evaluation/outcomes
		peutic regimen	medication, strength, changes in the prescribed dose and pattern of BP levels if records are available (e.g. Nifedipine / dose, route / sedatives, etc.)	planning and implementing relevant care	the relevant outcomes
		(Ref BP records)	• Record the BP of the client and maintain BP chart	Provides a clear picture for monitoring and	

Sl no	Date	Time	BP	Units	Rem	Sig

Contd...

Contd...

<table>
<tr><th>Subjective/ objective data</th><th>Nursing diagnosis</th><th>Objective</th><th>Interventions</th><th>Rationale</th><th>Evaluation/outcomes</th></tr>
<tr><td></td><td></td><td></td><td>• Educate and encourage the client to regularly take the prescribed meditation</td><td>maintaining BP</td><td></td></tr>
<tr><td></td><td></td><td></td><td>• Maintain drug chart as follows:
<table><tr><th>Sl no</th><th>Date</th><th>Drug</th><th>Dose</th><th>Time</th><th>Y/N</th><th>Rem</th><th>Sig</th></tr><tr><td></td><td></td><td></td><td></td><td></td><td></td><td></td><td></td></tr></table></td><td>Helps in maintaining BP within acceptable range</td><td></td></tr>
<tr><td></td><td></td><td></td><td>• Explain on the consequences over / and under dosage</td><td>Helps in monitoring the adhe-</td><td></td></tr>
</table>

Contd...

Contd...

Subjective/ objective data	*Nursing diagnosis*	*Objective*	*Interventions*	*Rationale*	*Evaluation/outcomes*
		Dietary management	• Assess the dietary pattern and food habits of the client	rence to the prescriptions	
			• Perform 24 hrs recall		
			• Calculate the actual Kcal, CHO, Fat contents and compare with RDA	Helps in devising suitable diet	
			• Devise a sample menu plan / (low cost diet) according to the lifestyle of the client		
			• Educate on the foods to be included and	Helps the client in	

Contd...

Contd...

Subjective/ objective data	*Nursing diagnosis*	*Objective*	*Interventions*	*Rationale*	*Evaluation/outcomes*
			foods to be avoided • Prepare a list of the above and give it to the client	avoiding items that elevate BP	
			• Advice specifically on the importance of low fat, low salt diet	Increased salt consumption increases BP A High fat diet increases the risk of developing athenosclerosis,	

Contd...

Contd...

Subjective/ objective data	*Nursing diagnosis*	*Objective*	*Interventions*	*Rationale*	*Evaluation/outcomes*
				further can elevate BP	
		Exercise and Sleep	• Advice and encourage regular exercises	Regular exercises increase LDH, which helps in maintaining the BP promotes cardiac well being	
			• Advice and educate on the importance of	Since body	

Contd...

Contd...

Subjective/ objective data	*Nursing diagnosis*	*Objective*	*Interventions*	*Rationale*	*Evaluation/outcomes*
			regular sleep (If required prescribe sedatives along with antihypertensives)	is at rest the sleeping BP is low	
		Health Education	Health educate the client on the following	Helps client in participating in self care	
			• Importance of regular intake of drugs • Dietary management	Helps in appropriate management of emergencies	

Contd...

Contd...

Subjective/objective data	*Nursing diagnosis*	*Objective*	*Interventions*	*Rationale*	*Evaluation/outcomes*
			• Exercise and sleep • S/S of hypo- and hypertension • Recognizing and management of hypo- and hypertension • Any other as relevant to the client		

CHAPTER 19

Guidelines for Write-up Formats—Practical Exam

COMMUNITY HEALTH NURSING

Heading to be included

1. Client/Beneficiary Name
2. Address
3. Family Profile
4. Socioeconomic Profile
5. House/Residence (Floor Plan)
6. Classification of Beneficiary
   - Newborn
   - Infant
   - Toddler
   - Preschooler
   - School going child
   - Antenatal mother
   - Postnatal mother
   - Adult/elderly with morbidity conditions
7. Physical Assessment/specific assessment according to the client
8. 24 hrs Recall
9. 24 hrs Recall Assessment with RDA/Sample menu
10. Specific Assessment – (depending on beneficiary)
11. Needs/Problem/Nursing Diagnosis list with priority
12. Nursing Care Plan
13. Health Education follow up and continuity care

WRITE-UP FORMAT FOR PRACTICAL EXAMINATION IN DETAIL

i. **Name of the Head of the Family**

House number :
Type of family :
Size of the family :
Religion :
Mother tongue :

ii. **Family Details**

S. No.	*Name of the family members*	*Relation-ship with head of the family*	*Age*	*Sex*	*Education*	*Occupation*	*Income*	*Marital status*	*Health status*

19

iii. **Socioeconomic Profile**

RISK STATUS	:	High Risk/ Normal	Village Name	:
Status of the family	:	Nuclear/ Joint/ Extended	Sub Centre	:
Religion		Hindu/ Christian/ Muslim	PHC	:
Area	:	Urban/Rural		

1.	Housing : own/rental		No. of living rooms :
	Type of house	:	Kutcha/Pucca/ Semipucca
2.	Ventilation	:	Adequate/Inadequate Artificial Resource : Fan/ Other Natural Resources
		:	Window to Window/ Window to Door/Door to Door
3.	Lighting	:	Adequate/Inadequate Sources : Electricity/Gas Lamp
4.	Kitchen	:	Separate/Inside the Room/Outside Size : Adequate/ inadequate Fuel Use : Kerosine/Fire wood/Cow dung/Gas/ Electricity
5.	Drainage	:	Open/Closed/Nil Cleanliness : Clean/ Dirty

Contd...

Contd...

6.	Water Supply	:	Adequate/Inadequate Sources : Well/Tap/ Bore well Storage : Hygienic/ Unhygienic
7.	Lavatory	:	Present/Absent : if Present Type : Sanitary/ Insanitary
8.	Refuse Disposal Collection		Hygienic/Unhygienic Disposal : Dumping/ Burrying/Burning
9.	Surrounding	:	Clean/Untidy
10.	Maternal and Child Healthservices		Eligible couples : Family Planning method adopted : No. of under fives : Immunization of Under Five : Immunized/Partially immunized/Not immunized

iv. **Physical Examination**

Sl. No.	*Item/Criteria*	*Parameter*	*Findings*
1.	Vital signs	Temperature Pulse Respiration Blood pressure	

Contd...

Contd...

Sl. No.	*Item/Criteria*	*Parameter*	*Findings*
2.	General appearance Mental status	Look Thin/Moderate/ Obese/Active/Alert/ Dull	
3.	Anthro-pometric measurement	a. Height b. Weight c. Head circumference d. Chest circumference e. Midarm circumference	
4.	Head	f. Scalp : clean/ dandruff g. Hair : flag sign/ easily pluckable/ lice /normal	
5.	Eyes	h. Eyelids – sty/ normal i. Conjunctiva : pale pink j. Presence of Bitot spots k. Xerophthalmia l. Discharge/squint/ normal	
6.	Ears	m. Otorrhoea/HOH n. Cerumen/Normal	
7.	Nose	o. Rhinorrhea/polyps p. DNS/Normal	

Contd...

Contd...

Sl. No.	*Item/Criteria*	*Parameter*	*Findings*
8.	Throat and Mouth	q. Lips – Cracked/ Angular Stomatitis/ Normal r. Gums – Gingivitis/ Bleeding/Normal s. Teeth – caries/ Missing tooth/ changes in enamel/ normal t. Tongue – Fissured/ Geographic tongue/Glossitis/ Normal etc. u. Tonsil – Enlarged/ Normal	
9	Neck	v. Lymph nodes – Enlarged/Normal w. Range of motion x. Enlargement of Thyroid gland	
10	Chest	Shape of chest Chest movement Lung sound Heart sound Breast	
11	Abdomen	Observation Palpation	

Contd...

Contd...

Sl. No.	*Item/Criteria*	*Parameter*	*Findings*
		Percussion Auscultation	
12	Extremities		
13	Genitalia		
14	CNS reflexes		

Reflexes (for infant and U5)

Sl. No.	*Name of the reflexes*	*Type*	*Present*	*Absent*	*Remarks*
1	Face	Blinking Corneal reflex Papillary reflex Doll's eye's reflex Glabellar reflex Sneeze reflex			
2.	Mouth and throat	Sucking reflex Gag reflex Rooting reflex Extrusion reflex			

Contd...

Contd...

Sl. No.	*Name of the reflexes*	*Type*	*Present*	*Absent*	*Remarks*
3.		Cough reflex Yawning reflex			
4.	Extremities	Great (palmar and plantar reflex) Babinski reflex			
5.	Motor	• Moro • Startle • Asymmetric tonic neck reflex • Reflex righting • Trunk incurvation reflex Dance or stepping reflex Crawling, playing reflex and toddler			

Contd...

Contd...

Sl. No.	*Name of the reflexes*	*Type*	*Present*	*Absent*	*Remarks*
6.	Deep tendon reflex	• Biceps, Triceps, Brachio-radialis patellar, Achilles reflex			

v. **Nutrition**

a. 24 hrs Recall (General)

Sl	*Time*	*Item*	*Qty.*	*CHO*	*Protein*	*Fat*	*Kcal*	*Iron*	*calcium*

b. 24 hrs Recall assessment

Sl No.	*Actual*	*RDA*	*Inference*
1.	CHO		
2.	Calorie		
3.	Fat		
4.	Calcium		
5.	Iron		

c. Sample menu

Sl No.	*Time*	*Item*	*Qty.*	*CHO*	*Pro.*	*Fat*	*Kcal*	*Iron*	*Calcium*

vi. **Specific Assessment of the Beneficiary**
vii. **Needs and Problems List Priority**
viii. **Nursing Diagnosis List and Priority**
ix. **Nursing Care Plan**

Sl. No.	*Diag-nosis*	*Objective*	*Plan of Implemen-tation*	*Evaluation*

x. **Health Education**
xi. **Continuity Care**

UNDER FIVE ASSESSMENT—GENERAL (COMMUNITY ORIENTED)

Assessment (Newborn/Infant/Preschool/School)

1. Place of birth – Home/Institution
2. Delivery conducted by – Untrained Dai/Trained personnel
3. Birth weight :
4. Apgar/Condition at birth
5. Any other relevant information

Physiological Parameters

1. Height 2. Weight 3. Head circumference 4. Chest circumference 5. MAC 6. Deworming 7. Vitamin 'A' 8. Pulse polio immunization	

DEGREE OF MALNUTRITION

$$\text{Gomez Classification} = \frac{\text{Actual weight}}{\text{Expected Weight}} \times 100$$

DEVELOPMENTAL MILESTONES

Sl. No.	*Milestone (Motor Dept.)*		*Achie-ved/Yes*	*No*	*Remarks*
	Age	*Motor*			
1.	3 Months	Holds head erect	Yes	No	
2.	6-8 Months	Sits with support	Yes	No	
3.	9-10 Months	Crawling	Yes	No	
4.	10-11 Months	Stands with sup-port	Yes	No	
5.	12-14 Months	Walks wide base	Yes	No	
6.	18-21 Months	Walks narrow base	Yes	No	
7.	24 months	Runs	Yes	No	

IMMUNIZATION

Sl. No.	*Age in months*	*Immunization*	*Yes*	*No*	*Remarks*
1.	At birth	BCG, 'O' Polio			
2.	1 ½ months	OPV_1, DPT_1			
3.	2 ½ months	OPV_2, DPT_2			
4.	3 ½ months	OPV_3, DPT_3			
5.	9 months	Measles & Vit A			
6.	1 ½ years	OPV_4, DPT_4 Booster			
7	5 years	DT			

- Include others till 16 years as relevant
- Ref. Immunization Schedule

19

DEWORMING : Every six month after one year

Sl No.	Age	Yes	No

VIT 'A' PROPHYLAXIS : Nine month to Five years/every 6 months

Sl No.	Age	Yes	No

U5 SPECIFIC ASSESSMENTS

NEWBORN ASSESSMENT

IDENTIFICATION DATA

Name :
Chronological age :
Developmental age :

Sex :
I P No./ward :
Address :
Diagnosis :
Date of admission :

Anthropometric Measurements

Measure-ment	*Book picture*	*Child picture*	*Remarks*
Head circum-ference			
Chest circum-ference			
Weight			
Height			

Vital Signs

Parameter	*Book picture*	*Child picture*	*Remarks*
Temperature			
Heart rate			
Respirations			
Blood pressure			

Sequence	*Items to be Observed*	*Remarks*
GENERAL APPEARANCE		
Body built	Mesomorphic/Endomorphic/ Ectomorphic	
Colour	Dark/Fair/Cyanosis/Pallor	
Posture	Normal/Abnormal (specify)	
Activity	Dull/Lethargic/Active	
SKIN		
Colour	Cyanosis/pink/bright red/ jaundice/pallor	
	Dryness/Flaking/Wrinkling	
Texture	Vernix caseosa/Lanugo/ Edema	
Skin lesion	Mongolian spots/milia/ Erythema	
HEAD TO FOOT EXAMI-NATION		
HEAD		
Size of the head	Microcephaly/macro-cephaly/hydrocephalus	
Hair	Color/distribution	
Scalp	Birth injury/cephalhematoma/ caput succedaneum	
Fontanelle suture	Anterior/posterior/size/ shape/wide sutures	

Contd...

Contd...

Sequence	*Items to be observed*	*Remarks*
EYES:	Colour/Eyebrows/ Eyelashes/Eye discharge/ Congenital anomalies/ blinking/papillary reaction	
NOSE:	Nasal polyp/DNS nasal discharge	
EAR:	Position of the pinna/ ecoiling/ear discharge/ wax/hearing capacity	
MOUTH AND THROAT		
Lips	Colour/condition/cleft lip/ palate	
Tongue	Colour/condition/congenital anomaly (micro/macrognathia)	
Teeth	Natal teeth	
Throat and pharynx	Redness/Epstein pearls/ absent or minimal salivation	
Neck	Movements/wry neck/ clavicles/lymph node	
CHEST:		
Thorax	Shape/symmetry expansion/posture	
Respirator sound	Sight/swish/rustle/ wheezing/rales	

Contd...

Contd...

Sequence	*Items to be observed*	*Remarks*
Heart	Size & location/cardiac murmurs	
Breast	Enlargement/twitches milk secretions/wide spaced nipples	
Lungs	Respiratory rate	
Heart	Heart rate/sound	
ABDOMEN:		
Inspection	Shape/size/condition of the cord/visible peristaltic waves/veins	
Auscultation	Bowel sounds	
Palpation	Liver margins/ palpable spleen/ tenderness/umbilical/ inguinal hernia/femoral pulses	
Percussion	Presence of gas/fluid or masses	
GENITALIA:		
Female	Labia & condition/ pseudomenstruation absence of vaginal opening/fused labia/ ambiguous genitalia	
Male	Urethral/anal opening/ undescended testes/	

Contd...

Contd...

Sequence	*Items to be observed*	*Remarks*
	phimose/hypospadiasis/ epicardia/hydrocoele/ ambiguous genitalia	
EXTREMI-TIES:	Symmetry/range of motion/polydactyly/ syndactyly/club foot/ hip dislocation/latex deep crease	
BACK / SPINE :	Spinal curves/spina bifida	
NEURO-MUSCULAR SYSTEM:	Hypotonic/Hypertonic/ Asymmetric posturing/ Tremors/Twitches	
REFLEXES:		
Eyes	Blinking/corneal/ papillary/Doll's eye	
Nose	Sneeze/Glabellas	
Mouth and Throat	Sucking/Gag/Rooting/ Extrusion/Yawn/Cough	
Extremities	Grasp/Babinski/Ankle Clonus	
Mass	Moro/Startle/Perez/ Asymmetric tonic neck/ Trunk incurvation/dance or step/crawl/placing	

ASSESSMENT INFANT (1 MON – 1 YR)

IDENTIFICATION DATA

Name :
Chronological age :
Developmental age :
Sex :
I P No./ward :
Address :
Diagnosis :
Date of admission :

ANTHROPOMETRIC MEASUREMENTS

Measurement	*Book Picture*	*Child Picture*	*Remarks*
Head circum-ference			
Chest circum-ference			
Weight			
Height			

Vital Signs

Parameter	*Book picture*	*Child picture*	*Remarks*
Temperature			
Heart rate			
Respirations			
Blood pressure			

Sequence	*Items to be observed*	*Remarks*
GENERAL APPEARANCE		
Body built	Mesomorphic/ Endomorphic/ Ectomorphic	
Color	Dark/Fair/Cyanosis/ Pallor	
Posture	Normal/Abnormal (specify)	
Activity	Dull/Lethargic/Active	
SKIN		
Color	Cyanosis/Pink/Bright red/ Jaundice/Pallor	
Texture	Dryness/Flaking/ Wrinkling	
Skin lesion	Erythema/Edema/Rashes/ Allergy	
HEAD TO FOOT EXAMINATION: HEAD		
Hair	Color/distribution	
Scalp	Injury/Scar/Clean/ dandruff/pediculosis	
Fontanelle suture	Closed/opened	
Fare	Pale/flushed puffiness/ fatigue/fear/anxious	

Contd...

Contd...

Sequence	*Items to be observed*	*Remarks*
EYES :		
Eyebrows	Normal or absent	
Eyelashes	Infection/sty	
Eyelids	Oedema/lesions/ ectropion/entropion	
Eyeball	Sunken or protruded	
Conjunctiva	Pale/red/purulent	
Sclera	Jaundice	
Pupils	Dilated, constricted, reaction to light	
Lens	Opaque or transparent	
Eye muscles	Strabismus	
EARS :		
External ear	Discharges, cerumen obstructing the ear passage location of pinna	
Tympanic membrane	Perforations, lesions, bulging	
Hearing acuity	Normal/deaf	
NOSE		
External nares	Crusty or discharge	
Nostrils	Inflammation of the mucous membrane, septal deviations	
MOUTH AND PHARYNX:		
Lips	Redness, swelling, crusted,	

Contd...

Contd...

Sequence	*Items to be observed*	*Remarks*
	cyanosis, angular, stomatitis/cleft lip/ fissures/oral thrush	
Odour of the mouth	Foul smelling	
Teeth	Appearance of temporary teeth/discoloration teeth decay	
Gums	Pale/bluish/bright red/ hypertrophy/bleeding hyperplasia/atrophy/ scorbutic gums	
Oral muscles membrane	Pale/bluish/yellow/milky white/swollen redness/ bleeding	
Tongue	Muroglossia/ microglossia/parrot tongue/tongue tie/ pale/dry/coated/pallers/ protrude	
Throat and pharynx	Enlarged tonsils redness, pus collection	
NECK		
Lymph nodes	Enlarged/palpable	
Thyroid gland	Enlarged	
Range of motion	Flexion/extension/ rotation/wrynelle/short neck	

Contd...

Contd...

Sequence	*Items to be observed*	*Remarks*
CHEST		
Thorax	Shape/symmetry of expansion/posture	
Breather sounds	Sigh/swish/rales/ wheeze/crepitus	
Heart	Size & location, cardiac murmur	
Breast	Enlarged	
ABDOMEN		
Observation	Skin rashes, scar, hernia, ascites, distension	
Auscultation	Bowel sounds	
Palpation	Liver margin/spleen/ tenderness/hernial	
Percussion	Presence of gas, fluid or masses	
EXTREMITIES	Movement of joint, tremors, clumbing of tinges, ankle edema/congenital anomalies. Spina bifida/curves	
BACK AND SPINE:	Patency of urethral/rectal opening	
GENITALIA AND RECTUM:	Inguinal lymph gland enlargement/vaginal discharge STD/congenital anomalies	

Contd...

Contd...

Sequence	*Items to be observed*	*Remarks*
REFLEXES		
Eye	Blinking/corneal/ papillary/doll's eye	
Nose	Sneeze/glabellas	
Mouth and Throat	Sucking/gag/rooting/ extrusion/yawn/cough	
	Grasp/Babinski/ankle clonus	
Extremities Mass	Moro/startle/perez/ asymmetric tonic neck/trunk incurvation/dance or step/ crawl/placing	

NOTE :

To calculate the weight of a child =

$$3\text{-}12 \text{ months} = \frac{\text{Age in month} + 9}{2}$$

ASSESSMENT TODDLER (1-3 YEARS)

IDENTIFICATION DATA

Name :

Chronological age :

Developmental age :

Sex :

I P No./ward :

Address :

Diagnosis :

Date of admission :

Anthropometric Measurements

Measurement	*Book Picture*	*Child Picture*	*Remarks*
Head circumference			
Chest circumference			
Weight			
Height			
Midarm circumference			

Vital Signs

Parameter	*Book picture*	*Child picture*	*Remarks*
Temperature			
Heart rate			
Respirations			
Blood pressure			

Sequence	*Items to be observed*	*Remarks*
GENERAL APPEARANCE		
Body built	Mesomorphic/Endomorphic/Ectomorphic	
Color	Dark/Fair/Cyanosis/Pallor	
Posture	Normal/Abnormal (specify)	
Activity	Dull/Lethargic/Active	
SKIN		
Color	Cyanosis/Pink/Bright red/Jaundice/Pallor	
Texture	Dryness/Flaking/Wrinkling	
Skin lesion	Erythema/Edema/Rashes/Allergy	
HEAD TO FOOT EXAMINATION : HEAD		
Hair	Color/distribution	
Scalp	Injury/Scar/Clean/dandruff/pediculosis	
Fontanelle	Closed/opened	
suture	Pale/flushed puffiness/fatigue/fear/anxious	

Contd...

Contd...

Sequence	*Items to be observed*	*Remarks*
EYES		
Eyebrows	Normal or absent	
Eyelashes	Infection/sty	
Eyelids	Oedema/lesions/ectropion/entropion	
Eyeball	Sunken or protruded	
Conjunctiva	Pale , red. Purulent	
Sclera	Jaundice	
Pupils	Dilated, constricted, reaction to light	
Lens	Opaque or transparent	
Eye muscles	Strabismus	
EARS		
External ear	Discharges, cerumen obstructing the ear passage location of pine	
Tympanic membrane	Perforations, lesions, bulging	
Hearing acuity	Normal/deaf	
NOSE		
External nares	Crusty or discharge	
Nostrils	Inflammation of the mucous membrane, septal deviations	

Contd...

Contd...

Sequence	*Items to be observed*	*Remarks*
MOUTH AND PHARYNX		
Lips	Redness, swelling, crusted, cyanosis, angular, stomatitis/ cleft lip/fissures/oral thrush	
Odour of the mouth	Foul smelling	
Teeth	Appearance of tempo-rary teeth/discoloration teeth decay	
Gums	Pale/bluish/bright red/ hypertrophy/bleeding hyperplasia/atrophy/ scorbutic gums	
Oral muscles membrane	Pale/bluish/yellow/ milky white/swollon redness/bleeding	
Tongue	Muroglossia/micro-glossia/parrot tongue/ tongue tie/pale/dry/ coated/pallers/protrude	
Throat and pharynx	Enlarged tonsils redness, pus collection	
NECK		
Lymph nodes	Enlarged/palpable	
Thyroid gland	Enlarged	
Range of motion	Flexion/extension/ rotation/wryneck/ short neck	

Contd...

Contd...

Sequence	*Items to be observed*	*Remarks*
CHEST		
Thorax	Shape/symmetry of expansion/posture	
Breather sounds	Sigh/swish/rales/wheeze/ crepitul	
Heart	Size and location, cardiac murmur	
Breast	Enlarged	
ABDOMEN		
Observation	Skin rashes, scar, hernia, ascites, distension	
Auscultation	Bowel sounds	
Palpation	Liver margin/spleen/ tenderness/ hernial	
Percussion	Presence of gas, fluid or masses	
EXTRE-MITIES:	Movement of joint, tremors, clumbing of tinges, ankle edema/congenital anomalies. Spina/bifida/curves	
BACK AND SPINE:	Patency of urethral/rectal opening	
GENITALIA & RECTUM:	Inguinal lymph gland enlargement/vaginal discharge STD/congenital anomalies	
BEHAVI-OURAL PROBLEMS	Temper tantrums/ Enuresis/Thumbsucking/ Nail biting/Pica/etc.	

NOTE :

To calculate the weight of a child =
1-6 years = Age in years × 2 + 8
Height = 2 to 12 years = Age in Year × 6 + 77

ASSESSMENT PRE SCHOOL (3-5 YEARS)

IDENTIFICATION DATA

Name :
Chronological age :
Developmental age :
Sex :
I P No./ward :
Address :
Diagnosis :
Date of admission :

Anthropometric Measurements

Measurement	*Book picture*	*Child picture*	*Remarks*
Head circumference			
Chest circumference			
Weight			
Height			
Midarm circumference			

Vital Signs

Parameter	*Book picture*	*Child picture*	*Remarks*
Temperature			
Heart rate			
Respirations			
Blood pressure			

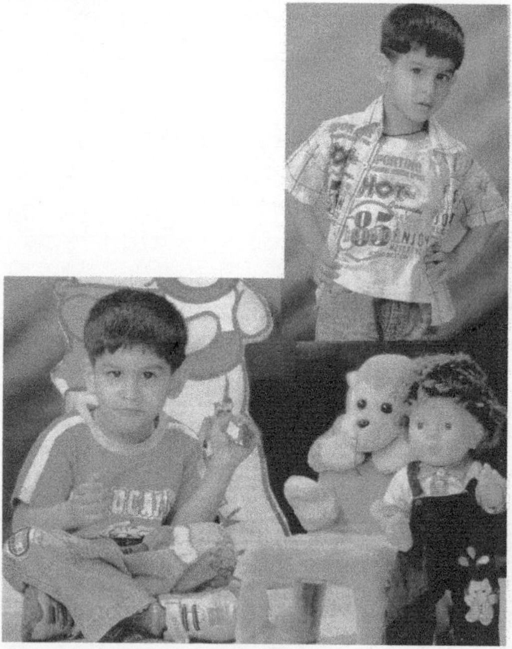

Assessment of School Going Child

Sequence	*Items to be observed*	*Remarks*
GENERAL APPEARANCE		
Body built	Mesomorphic/Endomorphic/Ectomorphic	
Color	Dark/Fair/Cyanosis/Pallor	
Posture	Normal/Abnormal (specify)	
Activity	Dull/Lethargic/Active	
SKIN		
Color	Cyanosis/Pink/Bright red/Jaundice/Pallor	
Texture	Dryness/Flaking/Wrinkling	
Skin lesion	Erythema/Edema/Rashes/Allergy	
HEAD TO FOOT EXAMINATION: HEAD		
HEAD		
Hair	Color/distribution	
Scalp	Injury/Scar/Clean/dandruff/pediculosis	
Fontanelle	Closed/opened	
suture	Pale/flushed puffiness/fatigue/fear/anxious	

Contd...

Contd...

Sequence	*Items to be observed*	*Remarks*
EYES		
Eyebrows	Normal or absent	
Eyelashes	Infection/sty	
Eyelids	Oedema/lesions/ ectropion/entropion	
Eyeball	Sunken or protruded	
Conjunctiva	Pale , red. Purulent	
Sclera	Jaundice	
Pupils	Dilated, constricted, reaction to light	
Lens	Opaque or transparent	
Eye muscles	Strabismus	
EARS		
External ear	Discharges, cerumen obstructing the ear passage location of pinna	
Tympanic membrane	Perforations, lesions, bulging	
Hearing acuity	Normal/deaf	
NOSE		
External nares	Crusty or discharge	
Nostrils	Inflammation of the mucus membrane, septal deviations	

Contd...

Contd...

Sequence	*Items to be observed*	*Remarks*
MOUTH AND PHARYNX		
Lips	Redness, swelling, crusted, cyanosis, angular, stomatitis/cleft lip/ fissures/oral thrush	
Odour of the mouth	Foul smelling	
Teeth Gums	Appearance of temporary teeth/discoloration teeth decay	
Oral muscles membrane	Pale/bluish/bright red/ hypertrophy/bleeding hyperplasia/atrophy/ scorbutic gums	
Tongue Throat and pharynx	Pale/bluish/yellow/ milky white/swollon redness/bleeding Muroglossia/microglossia/parrot tongue/ tongue tie/pale/dry/ coated/pallers/protrude Enlarged tonsils redness, pus collection	
NECK		
Lymph nodes	Enlarged/palpable	
Thyroid gland	Enlarged	
Range of motion	Flexion/extension/ rotation/wryneck/short neck	

Contd...

Contd...

Sequence	*Items to be observed*	*Remarks*
CHEST		
Thorax	Shape/symmetry of expansion/posture	
Breather sounds	Sigh/swish/rales/ wheeze/crepitul	
Heart	Size & location, cardiac murmur	
Breast	Enlarged	
ABDOMEN		
Observation	Skin rashes, scar, hernia, ascites, distension	
Auscultation	Bowel sounds	
Palpation	Liver margin/spleen/ tenderness/hernial	
Percussion	Presence of gas, fluid or masses	
EXTREM-ITIES:	Movement of joint, tremors, clumbing of tinges, ankle edema/congenital anomalies. Spina/bifida/curves	
BACK and SPINE:	Patency urethral/ rectal opening	
GENITALIA & RECTUM:	Inguinal lymph gland enlargement/vaginal discharge STD/ congenital anomalies	
BEHAVI-OURAL PROBLEMS	Temper tantrum/ Enuresis/Thumbsuck-ing/Nail biting/Pica/etc.	

NOTE :

To calculate the weight of a child =
1-6 years = Age in years × 2 + 8
Height = 2 to 12 years = Age in Year × 6 + 77

ASSESSMENT SCHOOL (6-12 YEARS)

IDENTIFICATION DATA

Name :
Chronological age :
Developmental age :
Sex :
I P No./ward :
Address :
Diagnosis :
Date of admission :

Anthropometric Measurements

Measurement	*Book picture*	*Child picture*	*Remarks*
Weight			
Height			
Midarm circumference			

Vital Signs

Parameter	*Book picture*	*Child picture*	*Remarks*
Temperature			
Heart rate			
Respirations			
Blood pressure			

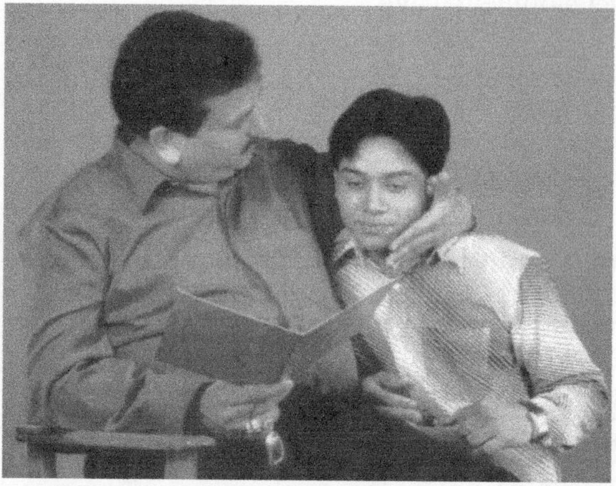

Assessment 6-12 Years

Sequence	*Items to be observed*	*Remarks*
GENERAL APPEARANCE		
Body built	Mesomorphic/ Endomorphic/ Ectomorphic	
Color	Dark/Fair/Cyanosis/ Pallor	
Posture	Normal/Abnormal (specify)	
Activity	Dull/Lethargic/Active	
SKIN		
Color	Cyanosis/Pink/Bright red/Jaundice/Pallor	
Texture	Dryness/Flaking/ Wrinkling	
Skin lesion	Erythema/Edema/ Rashes/Allergy	
HEAD TO FOOT EXAMI-NATION: HEAD		
Hair	Color/distribution	
Scalp	Injury/Scar/Clean/ dandruff/pediculosis	
Fontanelle	Closed/opened	
suture	Pale/flushed puffiness/ fatigue/fear/anxious	

Contd...

19

Contd...

Sequence	*Items to be observed*	*Remarks*
EYES		
Eyebrows	Normal or absent	
Eyelashes	Infection/sty	
Eyelids	Oedema/lesions/ ectropion/entropion	
Eyeball	Sunken or protruded	
Conjunctiva	Pale , red. Purulent	
Sclera	Jaundice	
Pupils	Dilated, constricted, reaction to light	
Lens	Opaque or transparent	
Eye muscles	Strabismus	
EARS		
External ear	Discharges, cerumen obstructing the ear passage location of pinna	
Tympanic membrane	Perforations, lesions, bulging	
Hearing acuity	Normal/deaf	
NOSE		
External nares	Crusty or discharge	
Nostrils	Inflammation of the mucous membrane, septal deviations	
MOUTH AND PHARYNX:		
Lips	Redness, swelling, crusted, cyanosis, angular, stomatitis/cleft lip/ fissures/oral thrush	

Contd...

Contd...

Sequence	*Items to be observed*	*Remarks*
Odour of the mouth	Foul smelling	
Teeth Gums	Appearance of temporary teeth/discoloration teeth decay	
Oral muscles membrane	Pale/bluish/bright red/ hypertrophy/bleeding hyperplasia/atrophy/ scorbutic gums	
Tongue	Pale/bluish/yellow/ milky white/swollon redness/bleeding Muroglossia/microglossia/parrot tongue/ tongue tie/pale/dry/ coated/pallers/protrude	
Throat and pharynx	Enlarged tonsils redness, pus collection	
NECK		
Lymph nodes	Enlarged/palpable	
Thyroid gland	Enlarged	
Range of motion	Flexion/extension/ rotation/wryneck/short neck	
CHEST		
Thorax	Shape/symmetry of expansion/posture	
Breather sounds	Sigh/swish/rales/ wheeze/crepitul	

Contd...

19

Contd...

Sequence	*Items to be observed*	*Remarks*
Heart	Size and location, cardiac murmur	
Breast	Enlarged	
ABDOMEN		
Observation	Skin rashes, scar, hernia, ascites, distension	
Auscultation	Bowel sounds	
Palpation	Liver margin/spleen/ tenderness/hernial	
Percussion	Presence of gas, fluid or masses	
EXTREMITIES:	Movement of joint, tremors, clumbing of tinges, ankle edema/congenital anomalies. Spina/bifida/curves	
BACK and SPINE:	Patency urethral/ rectal opening	
GENITALIA & RECTUM:	Inguinal lymph gland enlargement/vaginal discharge STD/ congenital anomalies	
BEHAVIOURAL PROBLEMS	Temper tantrum/ Enuresis/Thumbsucking/Nail biting/Pica/etc.	

NOTE :

To calculate the weight of a child =

$$7 - 12 \text{ Years} = \frac{\text{Age in year} \times 7 + 5}{2}$$

Height = 2 to 12 years = Age in year × 6+77

ANTENATAL ASSESSMENT

1. Antenatal Assessment

a. **General Information**
   a. Name
   b. Age
   c. Gravida/Parity
   d. LMP
   e. EDD
   f. Gestational age
   g. General investigation — Blood group/Typing/Hb%/VDRL, Scan, others
   h. Education occupation/income

b. **Physical Examination :** (including breast examination)

Criteria	*Observations*	*Findings*
Vital signs	Height	
Temperature	Weight	
Pulse	MAC	
Respiration	Chest circumference	
Blood pressure		
General	Thin/Moderate built	
Appearance	Obesity	
	Nourishment	

Contd...

19

Criteria	*Observations*	*Findings*
Head	Scalp : dandruff/ Hair : Flag/Easily Pluckable/Lice	
Eyes	Conjunctiva – pale/pink Presence of Bitot spots, Xerosis, Discharge/squint	
Ear	Otorrhoea/HOH/Cerumen	
Nose	Rhinorrhoea/Polyp/DNS	
Throat and Mouth	Lips gums (Incl. of teeth stated in Tongue general Tonsil assessment)	
Neck	Lymph nodes Range of Motion Enlargement of thyroid gland	
Chest	Shape of chest Chest movement Lung sounds Heart sounds Breast	
Abdomen	Observation/Inspection Auscultation Palpation Percussion Auscultation	
Extremities		
Genitalia		

(3a) AN PALPATION—VDRL/others - Scan

Obstetric Examination

Sl No.	*Examination*	*Criteria*	*Findings*
1.	Inspection	Size Contour Umbilicus Skin changes Fœtal movement Shape Flanks Bladder Previous scar	
2.	Palpation	Lateral paplation Left side Right side Lie Position Presentation No. of foetus Fundal palpation Fundal height Gestational age Abdominal girth	
3.	Pelvic palpation	GRIP – I GRIP – II (Pawlick's manoeuvre)	
4.	Auscultation	FHR	

POINTS TO BE REMEMBER

- Explain the procedure
- Arrange all the articles – bed side
- Advise the mother to empty the bladder
- Provide privacy
- Expose needed part
- Wash hands and warm up hands
- Stand at right side of the patient

FUNDAL PALPATION

- Start from the further side to nearer side
- Palpate with finger pads
- Identify the foetal part
- Movement of palpation should be from up to down

PELVIC PALPATION

GRIP I

- Stand facing the mother's feet

GRIP II

- Ask the mother to flex the knee
- With the help of right hand check the ballotment of head

AUSCULTATION

With the help of foetoscope assess the FHR

(3b) AN PALPATION- VDRL/others – Scan

Sl No.	*Month*	*Fundal height*	*Remarks*

4. **Iron Supplementation – Yes/No**
5. **Calcium - Yes/No**

Sl No.	*Month*	*Iron*	*Calcium*

6. **Weight Monitoring**

Sl No.	*Month*	*Weight*	*Remarks*	*Sign*

BP Monitoring

Sl No.	Month	B.P.	Remarks	Sign

7. Immunization

Sl No.	Month	T.T

8. Urine, Sugar and Albumin

Sl No.	Month	U/S	U/A	Remarks	Sign

9. 24 hrs recall (General)

Sl No.	*Time*	*Item*	*Qty*	*CHO*	*Pro.*	*Fat*	*Kcal*	*Iron*	*Calci.*

10. 24 hrs recall assessment

Sl No.	*Actual Intake*	*RDA*	*Inference*
	CHO		
	Protein		
	Fat		
	Calcium		
	Iron		

11. Sample Menu (low cost diet)

Sl No.	*Time*	*Item*	*Qty*	*CHO*	*Pro.*	*Fat*	*Kcal*	*Iron*	*Calci.*

12. Health Education (Items stated in overall assessment)

13. Follow up/Continuity Care

Health Education to Focus

1. AN registration and care
2. AN diet
3. Prevention of Infections
4. Iron/Calcium and Vitamin 'A' supplementations
5. Immunization
6. Preparation for delivery
7. Newborn Care/Immediate Postnatal Care
8. Family Planning
9. AN Exercises
10. Planned Parenthood

POSTNATAL ASSESSMENT

General Profile

a. Name
b. Age
c. Gravida/Parity
d. Date of Delivery
e. Place of Delivery : Home/Institution
f. Delivery Conducted by : Untrained/Trained Personnale

g. Type of Delivery : Natural/Assisted/ Caesarian
h. General Condition during delivery
  - TPR/BP
  - Breast/ Nipple condition

Vital Parameters

Sl No.	*Date/ Month*	*T.*	*P*	*R*	*BP*	*Involu-tion of of uterus*	*Lochia*

Specific Assessment

Sl No.	*Area*	*Criteria*	*Findings*
1.	Abdomen	Inspection Palpation Percussion Auscultation	
2.	Breast	Type of milk Secondary areola Warmness Tenderness of nipple	

Contd...

Contd...

Sl No.	*Area*	*Criteria*	*Findings*
		Cracked nipple	
		Sore nipple	
		Retracted	
3.	Abdomen	Fundal Ht	
4.	Perineum	Discharge	
	Lochia	Colour	
		Consistency	
		Odour	
5.	Extremities	Homan's sign	

Nutritional Assessment

- 24 hrs recall (as stated)
- Comparison of intake with RDA/In
- Sample menu in the following format

Sl No.	*Month*	*CHO*	*Protein*	*KCl*	*Fat*	*Calcium*	*Iron*	*Vit A*

Calcium/Iron/Vitamin – A supplementation

Health Education (as stated in Tabular Column format)

Follow Up Continuity Care

Health Education to focus on

1. Postnatal Care – Prevention of infection
2. Postnatal diet
3. Breast feeding – exclusive breast feeding, weaning and supplementary diet
4. New Born/Infant care – Growth Monitoring
5. Immunization
6. Contraception/Spacing/Family Planning
7. Postnatal Exercises
8. Home and Care of newborn

RECORDS REPORTS TO BE MAINTAINED IN RENDERING COMMUNITY HEALTH SERVICES RECORD FOR A DIABETIC CLIENT

Urine sugar chart

Sl No.	*Date*	*Urine Sugar*					*Inference*	*Sign*
		Blue	*Green*	*Yellow*	*Red*	*Brick Red*		

Drug Chart – Anti Diabetic drug

Sl No.	*Date*	*Time*	*Drug*	*Dose*	*Yes*	*No*	*Re-marks*	*Sign*

Insulin Chart

Sl No.	*Date*	*Time*	*Insulin*	*Units type*	*Yes*	*No*	*Re-marks*	*Sign*

Sample ID Card to be Carried Along

Name : *Age :*	*Blood Group :* *Medical Conditions :*	*Type :*	*Glucose Candy Diabetic*
Contact Person in case of emergency :			
Residential Add :			
Contact Number :			
Office Add :			

Sample Menu

Including foods to be included in plenty and to be avoided.

RECORDS PERTIENT TO HYPERTENSIVE CLIENTS

BP Chart

Sl No.	Date	Morning BP	Evening BP	Inference	Sig

Drug Chart

Sl No.	Date	Drug	Dose	Yes	No	Remarks	Sig

Sample

Diet with salt restricton including foods to be avoided and included in plenty.

RECORD RELEVANT FOR CLIENTS WITH COMMUNICABLE DISEASES – (TB, HANSENS), ETC.

Drug Chart

Sl No.	*Date*	*Drug*	*Dose*	*Yes*	*No*	*Remarks*	*Sig*

Focused Health Education

Points to be enlisted.

FAMILY CARE STUDY FORMAT

I. **INTRODUCTION**
II. **AREA MAP**
III. **SOCIOECONOMIC CONDITION**
- Name of the area
- Name of the taluk and district
- Population
- Information on social stratification
- Religion

- Education
- Occupation
- Total income of the family

IV. TRANSPORTATION AND COMMUNICATION

a. Type of road
   - Mud
   - Cement
   - Tar

b. Bus facility
   - BMTC
   - Private bus

c. Communication
   - Telephone
   - TV/Radio
   - Newspaper

V. GENERAL INFORMATIONS

1. Name of the family member
2. House number
3. Type of family
4. Religion
5. Caste
6. Mother tongue
7. Vital events

VI. FAMILY DETAILS

Sl No.	*Name of the family members*	*Relationship with head of the family*	*Age*	*Sex*	*Education*	*Occupation*	*Income*	*Marital status*	*Health status*

FAMILY TREE

VII. FLOOR MAP

VIII. ENVIRONMENTAL CONDITIONS

Criteria	*Observation*
A. HOUSING	
i. Type of House	
ii. Ownership	
iii. No. of rooms	
B. VENTILATION	
i. Type	
ii. No. of rooms	
iii. No. of windows	
C. ELECTRICITY	
D. WATER SUPPLY	
i. Well	
ii. Public Tap	
iii. Tank	
iv. Other sources	
E. KITCHEN	
i. Separate	
ii. Together/if joint family	
iii. Hand washing facility	
iv. Ventilation	
a. Window	
b. Chimney	
F. DISPOSAL OF WASTE	
i. Water	
a. open drainage	
b. soak pit	
ii. Refuse	
a. Composting	

Contd...

Contd...

Criteria	*Observation*
b. Burning	
c. Burial	
iii. Latrine :	
a. Yes	
b. No	
c. Open field defecation	
G. DOMESTIC ANIMALS	
i. Cattles	
ii. Poultry	
Others specify	

IX. FAMILY HEALTH ATTITUDES (Beliefs and Practices regarding)

a. Disease
b. Type of medical services
c. Physical defects
d. Maternal and child health
   - Antenatal
   - Delivery (intranatal)
   - Postnatal
   - Family planning
   - New born care
   - Immunization
   - Infant feeding

X. PHYSICAL EXAMINATIONS

Sl No.	Criteria	Finding
1.	**VITAL SIGNS** Temperature Pulse Respiration Blood pressure Height Weight	
2.	GENERAL APPEARANCE Nourishment Look Consciousness	
3.	Head Scalp Hair	
4.	EYES Eyebrows Eyelashes Eyelids Pupils Vision	
5.	EAR POSITION Discharge Hearing	
6.	NOSE Position Discharge Septum Sense of smell	

Contd...

Contd...

Sl No.	*Criteria*	*Finding*
7.	THROAT AND MOUTH	
	Lips	
	Gums	
	Teeth	
	Tongue	
	Tonsil	
8.	NECK	
	Lymph nodes	
	Range of motion	
	Enlargement of thyroid gland	
9.	CHEST	
	Shape of chest	
	Chest movement	
	Lung sound	
	Heart sound	
10.	ABDOMEN	
	Observation	
	Auscultation	
	Palpation	
	Percussion	
11.	EXTREMITIES	
12.	BACK	
13.	GENITALIA	
	INFERENCE :	

XI. NUTRITIONAL ASSESSMENT

Name :
Age :
Height
Weight
Occupation
Food habit
Dietary pattern
a. Staple food b. Number of meals c. Vegetable used d. Cooking practice e. Food storage

XII. (a) ASSESSMENT OF DIET

Sl No.	*Time*	*Menu*	*Amount*	*Calorie*	*CHO*	*Pro-tein*	*Fat Iron*	*Cal-cium*

XII. (b) COMPARISON WITH RDA

Sl No.	*Item*	*RDA*	*Actual consumption*	*Inference*
1.	CHO			
2.	PROTEIN			
3.	CALORIE			
4.	FAT			
5.	IRON			
6.	CALCIUM			

XII. (c) RECOMMENDED AS PER ICMR ALLOWANCES

Sl No.	*Time*	*Menu*	*Amount*	*Calorie*	*CHO*	*Protein*	*Fat*	*Iron*	*Calcium*

XIII. INFERENCE : Over all inference to be written

XIV. Add specific assessment depending on the beneficiary

XV. STUDY PLAN

Sl No.	Date	Duration	Procedure

XVI. NEEDS AND PROBLEMS WITH PRIORITY LIST

XVII. NURSING CARE PLAN

XVIII. HEALTH EDUCATION

XIX. SUMMARY

XX. CONCLUSION

House Hold Survey Schedule

1. House no. / Door No.:
2. Name of the Village :
3. Name of the street
4. Name of the head of the household
5. Name of the respondents
6. Religion
7. Caste
8. Type of house/hut/kutcha/pucca/own/rented
9. Mixed/seprated dwelling
10. Income per Annum : (T.H.H)

I. Particular of the house hold members

Sl.no.	Name of the house hold members	Relation to the head of the house hold	Age	Sex	Marital status	Educational status	Occupation	Income	Residential status	Immunization for US child											Vit A Droops No. of doses given	Folifer : No. of tablets taken	Morbidity				Others	Remarks
										DPT				MEASLES	OPV													
										BCG	I	II	III		0	I	II	III	Booster DPT	Booster OPV			Leprosy	Tuberculosis	Scabies	Nutritional Deficiency		

II Environmental Sanitation

1. Water supply: sources : tank: river: well: OHT : handpump — Adequacy : adequate/inadequate/protected/unprotected
2. Refuse disposal : open dumping/Burning/Manure pit
3. Waste water disposal : stagnation : yes/no
4. Excreta disposal : latrine : yes/no — If no, space available for construction : yes/no

Contd...

Sl No.	Name of the eligible couple	Age	Age of marriage	No of children born	Gender		Age of live children	No. of pregnancy	No of abortions	Emergency / reasons	Remarks of last Pregnancy	FP method adopted	Date of adoption	If discontinued date	Reasons for discontinuing	Reasons for non-adoption	EC priority	Remarks
					M	F												

Vital statistics

Sl No.	Name of the child	Name of parents	Sex	DOB	Place of birth	Attendance		Whether registered	Remarks	Sl no.	Name of the deceased	Age	Sex	Date of death	Place of death	Causes of death	Remarks

Surveillance for under 5 years / Adolescents & Women

Disease/complications	Name	Diagnosis	Investigation	Treatment	Referral
VPDS ADD/ARI RTI/STD Gynae problems Goiter					

NUTRITIONAL ASSESSMENT

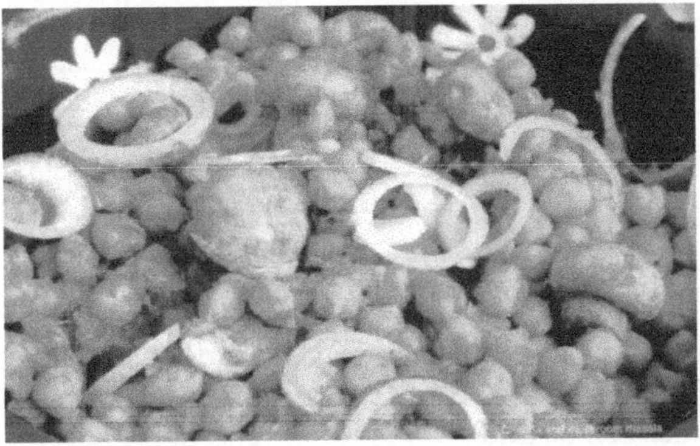

IDENTIFICATION DATA

Name :
Age :
Sex :
District :
Village :
Address :
Date :

ANTHROPOMETRIC ASSESSMENT

Height (cm)
Weight (kg)
Midarm Circumference (cm)
Head Circumference (cm)
Chest Circumference (cm)

$$\text{Degree of Malnutrition} = \frac{\text{Actual wt}}{\text{Expected wt}} \times 100$$

Between 70 and 79% of RWA – 1st degree Malnutrition

Between 60 and 69% of RWA – 2nd degree Malnutrition

< 60% of RWA – 3rd degree Malnutrition

< 50% if RWA – 4th degree Malnutrition

19

PHYSICAL EXAMINATION

Physical Examination	*Findings*
1. General appearance	Normal built/Thin built
2. Hair	Normal/Lack of Lusture/ depigmented/Thin
3. Face	Diffuse depigmentation/ Moon face

Contd...

Contd...

Physical Examination	*Findings*
4. Eyes	Conjunctiva : Normal/Dry/Wrinkled/Bitot's spot/Brown pigmentation/pale. Cornea : Normal/Dryness/Opaque
5. Lips	Normal/Angular stomatitis
6. Tongue	Normal/Pale/Red and raw/Flabby
7. Teeth	Caries
8. Gums	Normal/Spongy/Gingivitis
9. Glands	Thyroid enlargement/Parotid enlargement
10. Skin	Normal/Dry and scaly/dermatitis
11. Nails	Koilonychia
12. Extremities	Normal/Edematous/Congenital anomalies

NUTRITIONAL STATUS

a. Food-habits

Food-habits	Remarks
1. Vegetarian	
2. Non-vegetarian	

b. If non-vegetarian how often do you use:

c. 24 Hour Recall

Sl No.	*Time*	*Food Items*	*Qty. (Gms)*	*CHO (Gms)*	*Protein (Gms)*	*Fat (Gms)*	*Iron (mg)*	*Calcium (mg)*	*Calories (Kcal)*

COMPARISON OF RDA AND ACTUAL INTAKE

Sl No.	*Actual intake*		*RDA*	*Inference*
	CHO			
	FAT			
	PROTEIN			
	IRON			
	CALCIUM			
		Total	Inference	

19

MENU PLAN

Sl. No.	Time	Food Items	Qty (Gms)	Cho (Gms)	Protein (Gms)	Fat (Gms)	Iron (mg)	Vitamins			Calcium (mg)	Phosphorus (mg)	Calories (Kcal)
								A	B	C			

Index

A

B

E

F

G

H

I

M

N